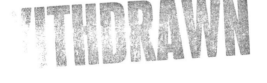

Patterns of Disease and Hunger

ANDREW LEARMONTH

Patterns of Disease and Hunger

David & Charles   Newton Abbot   London
North Pomfret (VT)   Vancouver

British Library Cataloguing in Publication Data

Learmonth, Andrew
    Patterns of disease and hunger. (Problems in
    modern geography.)
    1. Medical geography
    I. Title   II. Series
    616   RA792
    ISBN 0-7153-7538-5
Library of Congress Catalog Card Number 77-91741

Phototypeset in Times by Tradespools Limited Frome Somerset
and printed in Great Britain by
Biddles Limited Guildford
for David & Charles (Publishers) Limited
Brunel House Newton Abbot Devon

Published in the United States of America
by David & Charles Inc
North Pomfret Vermont 05053 USA

Published in Canada
by Douglas David & Charles Limited
1875 Welch Street North Vancouver BC

Contents

List of Figures

Introduction

Human geography includes the study of similarities and differences—and also trends over time—in population density in different parts of the globe. But sheer density, people per square mile or per square kilometre, is not a particularly meaningful measurement unless variations in level of life—or standard of living—can somehow be considered too. Levels of health and disease vary between places, and over time, and are relevant to such studies. The book could be subtitled *A Study in Medical Geography*, and it is intended to introduce the reader to some parts of this study of differences in health in different parts of the world. A selective treatment is justified in a one-man volume, for a single author can only see in part and prophesy in part, and also because a short and selective treatment should enable the reader to judge if he or she wants to go further, more deeply or more widely, into studies of this kind. The term medical geography is the one usually found in English to describe the geography of health and disease (and of health services too), the study of patterns of similarities and of differences between areas. (Working definitions of medical geography and a few other terms are given later in the introduction.)

Let us consider two examples of spatial patterns. Infant mortality is often taken as some indication of general levels of community health and well-being. Figure 1 shows that within a generally prosperous area like England and Wales there are marked differences, and that areas of high infant mortality are not randomly scattered, but concentrated in parts of the north and west of England and Wales. In broad regional patterns these differences are persistent, not just an accident of the particular run of years averaged for this particular map. Random local variations may also occur, but are not necessarily to be regarded

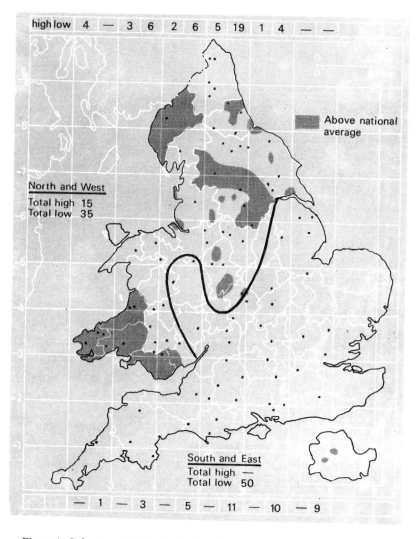

high low 4 — 3 6 2 6 5 19 1 4 — —

Above national average

North and West

Total high 15
Total low 35

South and East
Total high —
Total low 50

— 1 — 3 — 5 — 11 — 10 — 9

Figure 1. Infant mortality in England and Wales, 1954–58. Rates above the national expectation fall mainly in parts of the North and West region (see text), and in certain parts of London. The dots and figures refer to the statistical test known as χ^2. The particular sample here is not suitable for the test, but the totals strongly suggest that infant mortality is regionally concentrated in parts of our North and West region. (Source: Howe, G. M. *National atlas of disease mortality*, RGS/Nelson, 1970; Open University, *D203 Decision making in Britain*, Block 5, *Health*, Bletchley, Open University Press, 1972.)

so seriously. The broad pattern seems to reflect genuine differences in standards of health and health care and perhaps underlying differences in prosperity; most people will react with interest and concern and perhaps think that there is need for remedial action.

Figure 2 is different, showing the spread of a major regional epidemic of infectious hepatitis across south-eastern Australia; clearly there is a kind of epidemic wave that spread across some 400,000sq miles of country over a period of 2–3 years. This map is of interest, for itself and as an indication of how other epidemic waves may act, but one may also ask if any use can be made of such work. One answer is that if the spread and path of epidemic waves can be forecast, preventive or at least palliative action may be taken ahead of the wave of infection. If studies of disease can be linked with health services, they may indeed be of practical use as well as intellectual interest.

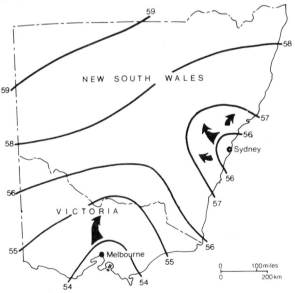

Figure 2. Sketch map of epidemic crest movement, Infectious Hepatitis, New South Wales, 1954–58. The isochrones or lines of equal timing (of passing of the crest of the epidemic wave) represent the year—54 = 1954, etc. Note that the time of the crest is succeeded, but especially preceded, by many occurrences of the disease. (Source: Brownlea, A. A., personal communication, 1968.)

The topic of the book, then, may well be interesting and important, but for what type of readership is it intended? The author is a professional geographer who has worked in this field for over 25 years, and thought about this book for over 5.

It is written with a largely student readership in mind, not so much as a textbook for examinations in human geography, but rather to introduce geographical ideas about an aspect of community life that may add a dimension to students' later work, in teaching, for instance. However, the book may bear some signs that it was first conceived for general readers with an interest in this particular geographical viewpoint on matters of life and death. The book may stimulate in a few readers the wish to engage in further study or research; if so, they will obviously have to go on to other deeper books, and I very much hope that the list of references will give such readers an entry point into a fascinating literature. My own concern with these studies has varied in emphasis over the years, and while I have of course tried to be up-to-date in the discussion, knowledge changes very rapidly in many of the fields covered. Readers for whom the latest advances in knowledge are important should start with the abstracting journals, like those, for instance, which are cited in the references at the end of the book, and then to journals recording advances in knowledge as they occur. Doctors interested in social and preventive medicine, nurses, health visitors and the like may find some interest in the book, but largely, I suspect, through looking at familiar material through geographical spectacles.

I have already suggested that a short book of this type must be selective. If too many diseases were discussed, the treatment would be so brief that the reader might be better to consult a medical encyclopedia. Moreover, it seems better to concentrate on topics where the geographical approach is particularly rewarding or enlightening in some way; where possible, examples have been chosen in which some advance in knowledge resulted, or even disease prevention or the potentiality of disease prevention. However, some indication of the scale of the problems discussed, in a world or countrywide perspective, will be given. There are gaps, too, owing to limitations in my own experience or reading: for example, I have not felt competent to include a chapter on the geography of mental illness, though I know that some of my geographer colleagues do interesting work in this field.

The book is more about the geography of disease than about the geography of health. Chapter 1 is concerned with the approach of the book, and contrasts health conditions in the developed as compared with the developing world. With examples, first for the developed world and then for the developing world, Chapters 2–4 review the geography of infectious disease, and Chapter 5 discusses non-infectious disease. Following a discussion of the geography of hunger (Chapter 6), Chapter 7 consists of case studies of the total impact of disease in particular areas, to show the way that a disease complex interacts with society. The geography of health services, though not a main concern of this book, is discussed in a short concluding chapter in which indications are given of further reading in this growing branch of the subject.

On rereading the manuscript of the book I have realized that both general and geographical readers may be impeded in reading the early chapters especially because of a few unfamiliar words, or words used in unfamiliar senses. To avoid this I am including here a number of working definitions that may save the reader trouble and delay.

Some working definitions

Bacteria: are microscopic single-celled vegetable organisms widespread in nature: for instance, in fermentation, decomposition of organic matter in the soil, and as normal constituents in the human intestinal tract. Some bacteria, however, cause human disease.

Endemic: constantly present (disease) in a particular population—the opposite of the more familiar *epidemic*. Epidemiology is the study of the behaviour of disease in populations, and has much in common with medical ecology. *Enzootic* and *epizootic* are corresponding terms for animal disease, and *zoonosis* for animal disease in which human beings become involved.

Medical ecology: the study of the web of relationships of a disease or a disease complex in its physical, biological and social environment. The *ecosystem* approach, following the pioneer ecologist Tansley, is to view a complex of organisms, plants and animals studied together in a particular site, and together with their whole habitat; the whole may be conceived as a set of interacting factors, in a system, the ecosystem, maintained in approximate equilibrium by the interactions.

Medical geography: the study of areal distribution patterns of (human) disease, preferably viewed as dynamic rather than static patterns, and aiming at explanation. The causation of the disease must be viewed from the viewpoint of the physiologist or the pathologist looking at the individual patient, but as important in this context is a social or community approach, and the approach of medical ecology.

Morbidity: the technical word for illness, from the original meaning of 'morbid', and corresponding to *mortality* for deaths.

Pandemic: an epidemic on the world scale.

Pathogen or pathogenic organism: a technical term preferred to 'germs' as the cause of infectious disease.

Viruses: originally and literally poisons, are technically much smaller organisms than bacteria, only visible since the invention of the electron microscope; many of them cause disease in plants and animals, including man.

CHAPTER ONE

Disease and Environment: A Spatial View

The introduction concluded with some working definitions of terms concerning certain relations between man, the environment and particular diseases. First in this chapter I would like to put some of these into action, as it were, in relation to yellow fever, a much dreaded disease 50 years ago and even today, and then to use the material on yellow fever as a basis in discussing the degree to which studies of man-disease relations are avoidably anthropocentric or man-centred, and how far unavoidably so.

Figure 3 shows that yellow fever is ultimately a disease of animals, a zoonosis—in fact a disease of monkeys. The yellow fever virus circulates between certain species of monkeys generally living at the main 'crown level' reached by the spreading tops (crowns) of equatorial rain-forest trees. The virus is carried from infected to susceptible monkeys by an insect 'vector', belonging to particular species of forest mosquitoes such as *Haemagogus* in Amazonia. These particular species are mosquitoes of the main crown layer of the forests adapted to that particular environment. The complex layered structure of equatorial rain forest produces not just one but a whole series of different environments; each has a different climate, or a different *micro*climate, to distinguish within the more general *macro*climate or 'large scale climate', which is often described as equatorial rain-forest climate. Monkeys, the virus and mosquitoes represent three components of a whole complex system of plants

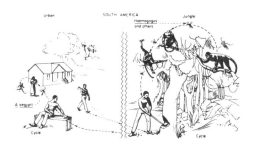

Figure 3. Jungle Yellow Fever. 'The drawing shows the manner of acquiring jungle yellow fever and the transmission of the virus from the forest to the man-mosquito cycle. The transmission by *Aëdes aegypti* is represented as occurring outside the house, whereas in all probability most of it takes place within doors. The broken lines indicate that the house may be some distance from the forest.' (Source: [including caption] Strode, G. K. [ed]. *Yellow fever*, New York, McGraw, 1951, Fig 62.)

and animals that co-exist, not in a static or completely unchanging set of relations, but fluctuating around some sort of equilibrium. These three elements happen to be the vital ones for the yellow fever cycle, but they belong to a wider complex, often called an ecosystem, as defined earlier. Note that man's activities form part of the system as well as those of different species of mosquitoes and of the yellow fever virus; in a lumbering community, we have to consider the movements of men, women and children in relation to the forest, but also as they go shopping in their market town and come into contact with urban mosquitoes, so that the virus and the yellow fever cycle can then be diffused along lines of communication and out into the populous and susceptible regions. The point of contact between man and the monkey disease of the rain forest provides one of the great stories of medical research; if a field medical team in eastern Colombia had not noticed a cloud of mosquitoes fly up from a felled giant tree, some of them biting lumbermen, the discovery of yellow fever as fundamentally a disease of rain-forest monkeys might never have been made—or might have been long delayed. Significant in itself, the new vistas of microclimate and microecology revealed have been stimulating in many other problems of man-environment relations.

This example should bring to life the earlier working definition of medical ecology, which is here concerned with a disease cycle, with a web of interrelations underlying that cycle, in a particular site—at the crown layer of a rain-forest area in Brazil.

In contrast medical geography is concerned with *area*, with spatial distribution. In Figure 4, a map of yellow fever throughout the world, the areal distribution pattern clearly suggests a tropical disease, though there have been historic invasions of sub-tropical and even temperate tracts, especially near seaports. This pattern was not fully understood, in fact it was misunderstood, until the ecology illustrated in Figure 3 was discovered in the 1930s. It was well enough known that in tropical towns and cities, and in extra-tropical seaports etc, the disease was carried from infected man to susceptible man by house-haunting mosquitoes, *Aëdes aegypti*, breeding successfully in urban waste water etc. It was then thought that the disease had three factors—the virus, man and *Aëdes aegypti*—and a major and costly crusade to wipe yellow fever from the globe was financed by the Rockefeller Foundation on that mistaken assumption.

To be fair, in the course of this campaign the true ecology of yellow fever became known, and it could be seen as a disease of

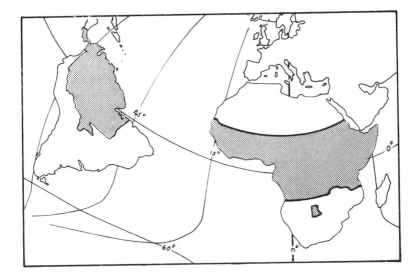

Figure 4. World Distribution of Yellow Fever, c 1950. (Source: May, J. M. 'Map of the world distribution of dengue and yellow fever', *Geog Rev*, 42, 1952, 283–6.)

monkeys, with a forest mosquito vector, into which man stumbles; once the virus is circulating in towns and cities, and moving along trade routes etc, the man/virus/*Aëdes aegypti* cycle does indeed come into its own. But the disease cannot be wiped out except by completely clearing the rain forests, and with them the small part of their ecology containing the monkey/virus/forest mosquito relations—an unthinkable procedure that would lead to many undesirable consequences. It can, however, be kept under control by carefully planned measures along the forest margins from which it used to sweep into the more populous parts of equatorial Africa and Latin America, and so out into the world's trade routes. An epidemic moving out from the forest into the towns and cities of Brazil is mapped in Figure 5.

This example may serve as a kind of working model to explain the relations between medical geography and medical ecology. The static or 'snapshot' map of a particular moment like Figure 4, and the dynamic map of movement like Figure 5, clearly link up with the disease cycle and the underlying network of movement and relationships of virus, monkey, mosquito and man of Figure 3. The areal distribution, on the ground or on the map, may sometimes give vital clues in the search for the ecological relations; nevertheless, the ecological is normally the key viewpoint in explanation, though surely in turn dependent on findings from pathology and microbiological laboratories.

The geography is always worth studying, for example, in relation to movements of disease from one environment to another—the 'exotic' disease, which is a serious problem in these days of rapid air transport—or again in relation to the strategy and logistics of the needs for men, money and material in a campaign of disease control or eradication. On the other hand, purely illustrative maps do have an educational role: they can communicate a great deal of information quickly—for instance, in spreading knowledge about the risks of importing exotic disease, like cholera in holidaymakers returning from Spain or northern Africa, or the apparently inexorable march of rabies across Europe at the time of writing.

Medical geography, then, deals with areal or spatial patterns of disease, which are described, often by using maps as an analytical

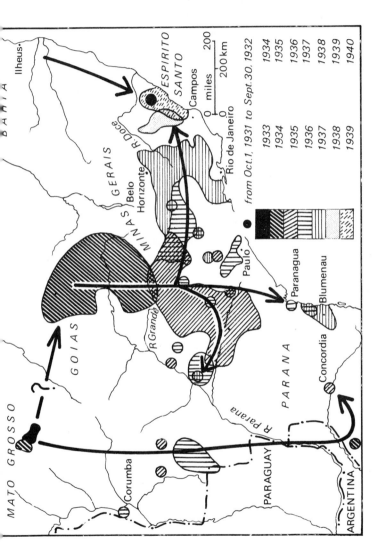

Figure 5. Probable route of spread of yellow fever epizootic of 1931–40 in Brazil, as indicated by chronological appearance of jungle yellow fever. (Source: [including caption] Strode, G. K. [ed]. *Yellow fever*, New York, McGraw, 1951, fig 52, Fig 52. Used with permission of McGraw-Hill Book Company.)

tool to break up a disease process into separate components for purpose of study, and so aid explanation. The medical geographer has to delve into a wide range of medical and biological literature, extending beyond the normal limits of geographical study into fields like medical ecology and epidemiology, as defined in the Introduction. But if the search for previous work proves negative, or reveals findings inconsistent with his own work, the medical geographer may have to be his own ecologist. Much medical geography might be a branch of biogeography, with biology as its sister science, and another part might be a branch of social geography, linked with sociology and other social sciences. Yet medical geography and medical ecology both include the word medical. What kind of legacy do they carry from the contact with medicine? Medicine has for millenia been founded on a particular ethic, including unwritten assumptions, originally founded on the Hippocratic oath, and though the oath's direct use has decreased in schools of medicine during the last few decades, it it still worth quoting to illustrate the spirit it aimed to invoke.

I swear by Apollo the physician, and by Asklepios, Hygeia, and Panacea and all the gods and goddesses, and call them to witness that I will keep this oath and contract to the best of my ability and judgement: to regard him who teaches me this art as equal to my own parents; to share my living with him, and provide for him in need; to treat his children as my own brothers, and teach them this art if they wish to learn it, without payment or contract; to give guidance, lectures, and every other kind of instruction to my own sons and those of my teacher, and to students bound by contract and oath to medical law, but to nobody else.

I will prescribe treatment to the best of my ability and judgement for the good of the sick and never for a harmful or illicit purpose. I will give no poisonous drug, even if asked to, nor make any such suggestion; and likewise I will give no women a pessary to cause abortion. I will both live and work in purity and godliness. I will not operate, not even on patients with stone, but will give way to specialists in this work. I will go into the houses that I visit in order to help the sick, and refrain from all deliberate harm or corruption, especially from sexual relations with women or men free or slave. Anything I see or hear about people, whether in the course of my practice or outside it, that should not be made public, I will keep to myself and treat as an inviolable secret. If I abide by this oath, and never break it, let all men honour me for all time on account of my life and work; but if I transgress and break my oath, let me suffer the reverse.

It is not too much to claim that the unwritten assumption is that the medical man must always accept that the saving of human life is invariably a good thing, so that medicine is almost by definition anthropocentric, centred on man. So is this book. Yet, paradoxically, clearer vision and deeper understanding are often attained by divorcing studies as far as possible from anthropocentrism. Consider an infection of human beings by an organism, a parasite. It may cause ill effects, or illness. If so, to a doctor, the infection is almost synonymous with disease, and he certainly views it in that light. If the infection does not cause disease, it is of no interest to a doctor as such, except perhaps as an indicator of general conditions of hygiene.

An example may clarify this issue. Two contrasted bacteria found in the human gut are *Salmonella typhi*, the organism causing typhoid fever; and *Escherichia coli*, which in comparatively rare cases causes kidney disease or peritonitis, especially in children or pregnant women, but is normally a harmless taken-for-granted part of one's intestinal flora, and so quite justly regarded as a commensal parasite—literally one sharing the same table! To a doctor *Salmonella typhi* is clearly a pathogen, a cause of illness, but *Escherichia coli* is generally of interest only as an indicator of pollution of water or food by human excreta, enough to alert him to the possibility of other intestinal parasites, including *Salmonella typhi*, in that particular community.

Let us abandon the professionally anthropocentric viewpoint of the medical man, and look at the same parasites through the eyes of a biologist. He also studies relations between parasites and host, but instead of harmless or pathogenic organisms, he will often treat the relation more objectively, simply as phenomena for study, as compared with the doctor. Thus the relations between *Salmonella typhi* and the people who are ill from it may be described as imperfect host-parasite adjustment, while there is near-perfect host-parasite adjustment between *Escherichia coli* and the vast majority of its human hosts.

At first sight it may seem merely an irritating academic quibble to fuss over the distinction between a parasite causing illness and one not causing it, the pathogenic and non-pathogenic, and on the other hand the concept of near-perfect as compared with imperfect host-parasite adjustment. But, as we shall see at various points in the book, the less anthropocentric viewpoint does enable the zoologist or zoologically minded epidemiologist more readily to see the picture whole, and not through anthropocentric spectacles. Of course to make the point I have almost caricatured the positions: medical scientists and many medical practitioners are as capable as the next man of adopting the more objective and non-anthropocentric viewpoint. One final note on *E. coli*: recently animal experiments strongly suggest that *E. coli* is more than merely commensal, and that the organism has a positive and important role in synthesizing vitamin K, an essential for the functioning of the liver and control of the clotting process in the blood.

To revert to the studies of yellow fever noted earlier, the problem of Figures 3–5 might well have been elucidated much earlier had the approach been less anthropocentric from the outset, and more aimed at understanding the whole web of relations between parasites and host. Later chapters will afford many illustrations of this.

One useful modern viewpoint is to view diseases, particularly infections, as man-environment flow systems, and Figure 16 applies this to malaria, where the idea of a cycle in the infection has been current since 1897, with its discovery by Sir Ronald Ross and independently by the Italian worker Grassi. The diagram does not aspire to represent any more than some sequences and relations in a much more complex total system; it is merely a conceptual framework—a framework of understanding—or simply one way of looking at the ecology of a disease.

One problem in the diagram used here is that the oval representing man is baldly divided into infected man and susceptible man. Within these simple tags are subsumed all the complexities of different occupations, of social groupings, of degrees of prosperity, of consciousness or perception of ill-health as a state to be remedied if possible, of different types of work in different places, with different sorts of journeys between home and work, and so on.

All these and other complexities can be viewed from the particular framework of analysis or understanding offered by geography. Accepting the definition given earlier, at least for the moment, this brings in area or space. So our main objective in medical geography is to study health when we can, but more often disease, since we can acquire data on it more easily; the analysis is to take account of medical ecology, of a web of relations straddling the physical and social networks, but in the search for areal patterns of health and disease. In a nutshell, and echoing the chapter title, we study disease and environment from a spatial viewpoint; we study a space-environment, biogeographic and socio-economic. We shall attempt this task in relation to both the developed world and the underdeveloped world, so the next section of this introduction is to discuss these terms.

The developed world is the world of high standards of material living under capitalist, communist or mixed economies, and very largely, too, the world of the 'consumer society' with until recently at least an ethos of ever-expanding aspirations to possess consumer goods of many kinds; these include many consumer durables—but with built-in obsolescence—making heavy demands on resources. These societies are industrialized, and many of them have passed through a phase of lower standards of material living, and (notably for the purposes of this book) poor standards of health, short expectation of life and so on. Britain during the Industrial Revolution can easily be over-dramatized as a place of dark satanic mills, urban slums, poverty and misery for the làbouring masses; but it did have, for instance, the terrible nineteenth-century epidemics of cholera, related very largely to poor conditions of water supply and sewage disposal, and equally a strong stimulus towards sanitary reform. Again the infant

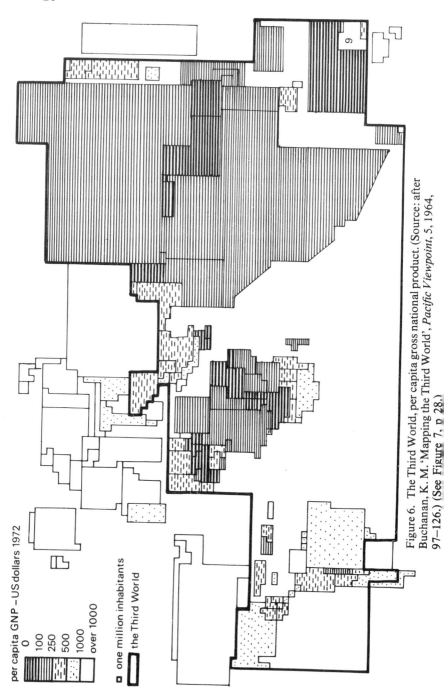

per capita GNP – US dollars 1972

0
100
250
500
1000
over 1000

□ one million inhabitants

▬ the Third World

Figure 6. The Third World, per capita gross national product. (Source: after Buchanan, K. M. 'Mapping the Third World', *Pacific Viewpoint*, 5, 1964, 97–126.) (See Figure 7, p 28.)

mortality rate in Great Britain as late as 1900 was about 145 per 1,000 live births, a figure somewhat higher than that for modern India. Thus it was only after the main Industrial Revolution period that Britain attained what we now think of as normal standards of health and health care.

The underdeveloped world is, conversely, the world of low standards of material living (Figures 6–7), of poverty, ignorance and ill-health. Many underdeveloped countries have become independent from former colonial masters in the developed world since World War II, and on the whole the new independent governments aim at raising standards of material living by planning their own industrial revolution while making radical improvements in health conditions. Commonly it proves easier to effect death control than birth control, and this era of ferment in the developing world, as it is sometimes hopefully called, is one of peculiar stresses. These now include a growing belief that the post-colonial world is one of exploitation of the developing by the developed world, almost as in colonial days; and a growing recognition that similar exploitation of poorer by richer areas of segments of the population can and does take place within developing countries—the Third World of some commentators, the others being the capitalist and the communist worlds. How does the interplay of independence, attempted industrialization, and aspirations towards radical improvement in health conditions affect our theme of the geography of disease?

The underdeveloped world has a much less complex technology than the developed, though this is by no means to say that its societies are simple. However, technology can be and is being imported. Some of the imported technology is elaborate, like the great steelworks in India, and the impact of many of the resultant industrial towns on the surrounding area has been disappointing. For this and other reasons there is a movement in favour of 'intermediate technology' rather than very sophisticated technology in many recent plans for economic development in Third World countries—that is, a level of technology more likely to be assimilable into the society as a whole and to act as a catalyst in producing an appropriate and self-sustaining development, rather than partially successful imitations of advanced,

28

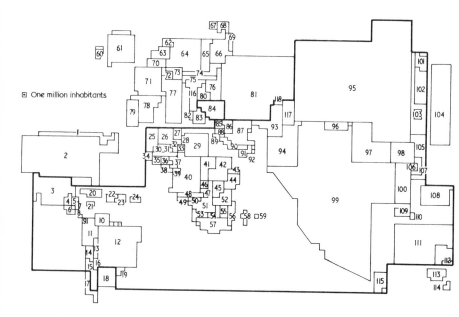

Figure 7. Location map and numerical index for Figure 6.

1 Canada; 2 United States; 3 Mexico; 4 Guatemala; 5 Honduras; 6 El Salvador; 7 Nicaragua; 8 Costa Rica; 9 Panama; 10 Venezuela; 11 Colombia; 12 Brazil; 13 Bolivia; 14 Ecuador; 15 Peru; 16 Paraguay; 17 Chile; 18 Argentina; 19 Uraguay; 20 Cuba; 21 Jamaica; 22 Haiti; 23 Dominican Republic; 24 Puerto Rico; 25 Morocco; 26 Algeria; 27 Tunisia; 28 Libyan Republic; 29 Arab Republic of Egypt; 30 Mauritania; 31 Mali; 32 Niger; 33 Chad; 34 Senegal; 35 Guinea; 36 Ivory Coast; 37 Ghana; 38 Liberia; 39 Togo; 40 Nigeria; 41 Sudan; 42 Ethiopia; 43 Somalia; 44 Kenya; 45 Uganda; 46 Rwanda; 47 Burundi; 48 Cameroon; 49 People's Republic of Congo; 50 Central African Republic; 51 Zaire; 52 Tanzania; 53 Angola; 54 Zambia; 55 Rhodesia; 56 Mozambique; 57 South Africa; 58 Malagasy Republic; 59 Mauritius; 60 Ireland; 61 United Kingdom; 62 Denmark; 63 Netherlands; 64 Federal Republic of Germany; 65 German Democratic Republic; 66 Poland; 67 Norway; 68 Sweden; 69 Finland; 70 Belgium; 71 France; 72 Switzerland; 73 Austria; 74 Czechoslovakia; 75 Hungary; 76 Romania; 77 Italy; 78 Spain; 79 Portugal; 80 Bulgaria; 81 USSR; 82 Albania; 83 Greece; 84 Turkey; 85 Lebanon; 86 Syrian Arab Republic; 87 Iraq; 88 Jordan; 89 Israel; 90 Saudi Arabia; 91 Yemen Arab Republic; 92 People's Democratic Republic of Yemen; 93 Iran; 94 Pakistan; 95 People's Republic of China; 96 Nepal; 97 Bangladesh; 98 Burma; 99 India; 100 Thailand; 101 Democratic Republic of Korea; 102 Republic of Korea; 103 Hong Kong; 104 Japan; 105 Vietnam; 106 Laos; 107 Khmer Republic; 108 Philippines; 109 Malaysia; 110 Singapore; 111 Indonesia; 112 Papua New Guinea; 113 Australia; 114 New Zealand; 115 Sri Lanka; 116 Yugoslavia; 117 Afghanistan; 118 Mongolia

particularly western, countries. Intermediate technology in health services may also be appropriate, not just second best, and the 'barefoot doctors' of China are often cited as an exemplar.

Some of the stresses in the Third World arise from very rapid changes linked with imported technology, and we shall see that even the population explosion itself may be an example of this. Since World War II much of the Third World has experienced a phase of decolonization. The newly independent countries have, naturally enough, given a high priority to tackling their most vulnerable problems of disease and hunger, with the encouragement and indeed active collaboration of the United Nations and other international agencies such as the World Health Organization. Concurrently, economic development has been attempted. Has our subject matter, and preoccupation with medical geography, caused us to put the cart before the horse here? Which did come first after independence, the aspirations towards economic development and higher standards of living, or health campaigns—directed in the first instance at death control, which, given the technology and human attitudes of recent decades, has been easier to accomplish than birth control? And which should come first? No doubt the drive towards economic development was built into the nationalist and anti-colonialist movements. Jawaharlal Nehru, for instance, was chairman of the Congress Party's committee on development planning a decade or more before independence was achieved; the revolution was largely one of rising expectation. But the accidents of history put health programmes into the forefront.

World War II, waged in such diverse climates and disease complexes, had brought great advances in medicinal drugs or chemotherapy, and especially in insecticides, including the so-called residual (or simply long-lasting) ones like DDT. Thus louse-borne typhus could be controlled by a vigorous campaign of dusting with DDT against body lice, and malaria could be controlled by a combination of prophylactic, or more strictly suppressive drugs like the wartime mepacrine, along with spraying DDT solutions over living quarters, workshops, stables, and shelters of all kinds, and so killing off resting adult mosquitoes (see also Chapter 4). The technology was such that great advances in disease control could be achieved with comparatively little collaboration from the people of the newly independent countries. (DDT would not of course now be applied over such wide areas of the world, because of the harmful effects of its spreading through the world ecosystem.) Economic development, on the other hand, was much more difficult to programme in any mechanical way, and has been proportionately more liable to disappointments and setbacks. Many stresses result from this fact.

At the same time as these developments in disease control were taking place there was a marked speeding up and greater ease of travel, and also in verbal communications of all kinds. These brought a quickening of world sensitivity and response to the problem of hunger. With wartime experience of better dietetic education, at least in some of the countries taking part in the war, notably Britain, came a more widespread awareness of malnutrition as a serious problem in addition to famine, sheer hunger, or more chronic manifestations of undernutrition (these distinctions are developed in Chapter 6).

The years since World War II are often thought of as the era of the population explosion. What is the relation, if any, between the so-called population explosion and the changing geography of disease and hunger?

There is a population explosion in the sense that in many countries the human population has for one or two decades now been rising sharply, between 2 and 3 per cent per annum, sometimes more. Some of the highest rates are in the underdeveloped world. They affect large absolute numbers, so that the underdeveloped world contained 2,000 million people in 1960 as compared with an expected total of 3,000 million in 1981. Yet the population explosion is not confined to the underdeveloped world. At least until recently many of the developed countries have been increasing population more sharply than they have in earlier decades this century; and, as has been pointed out, an individual in the developed world claims a much larger share of the world's resources than does a person in the underdeveloped world.

The part played in the population explosion by changes in disease patterns is debatable; the problem is discussed in relation to malaria in Chapter 4. Meanwhile we may regard health campaigns and the like as one cause among many of the upsurge in rates of population increase. Death rates have fallen sharply. Infectious diseases remain much more important in underdeveloped than in developed countries as causes of illness and death, but some of the most important are carried by insect vectors and have been particularly successfully controlled by residual insecticides in large and populous parts of the underdeveloped world. Infant mortality rates remain high compared with those in the developed world, but have fallen markedly in many underdeveloped countries during the last 20 years. Expectation of life at birth is rising, to resemble that, say, in England in 1901. Heart diseases and cerebral thrombosis, mainly diseases of the middle-aged and elderly, are less common in underdeveloped countries, probably because people do not live long enough to die from them. Cancers are common, but the sites vary for reasons by no means clear; cancer of the liver is important in many tropical countries and, locally, cancer of the oesophagus. In part these changes can be related to specific health measures and some of these have certainly had a crucial impact as a cause of change. But lowering of death rates and infant mortality rates is sometimes associated with general improvements in standards of living—with changes in social and economic conditions, rather than with specific health measures. Historically this was true of the retreat of malaria and of leprosy from western Europe, and much of the population explosion may be due to similar indirect causes of improvement.

Is there a vicious circle present? Does the population increase cause increased hunger and malnutrition? In places it almost certainly does—in some clearly overpopulated rural parts of India, for instance, as well as in the urban slum areas to which surplus population may be pushed by the pressures on landless labourers in the countryside, as in drought years. Some health campaigns, notably anti-malaria campaigns, may have increased human suffering rather than diminished it. Pressure to mount anti-malaria campaigns could not, should not have been resisted; it is not the fault of the malariologists. But these campaigns could and should have been accompanied by more strenuous, well planned and determined efforts to secure more, much more, economic development in the underdeveloped world than has in fact been successfully implanted as self-sustaining economic activity.

The responsibility no doubt lies mainly with the governments of the newly independent countries. After all, they *are* independent! But some share lies with the developed countries also. Probably the basis of accounting is too narrowly based. Aid for developing countries there has been, but too little, too piecemeal, too much concerned with how the donor country's interests can be served. It is certainly difficult to accept in the era of successful moon shots and lunar exploration that commensurate effort would not have secured better economic development programmes, and more than kept pace with the so-called population explosion until it eases off or is controlled.

Will population increase ease off in this way? There is at least some evidence, some of it dating as far back as the early 1950s, that better standards of living may reduce the pressures on people to have large numbers of children, since larger proportions may be expected to survive if the toll of hunger and disease is reduced.[1] More recently data from the state of Kerala in south-western India show the potential of substantial increases in age of marriage in slowing population growth.

In this chapter I have tried to set out some main themes of the book. They comprise the interesting web of relations of medical ecology, and the case for linking ecological studies with medical geography and spatial distributions; the advantages of minimizing anthropocentrism in approaching this field; the contrasts, commonalties and interactions between the developed and the developing world; and the implications of all these for studies of medical geography in a time of ferment and change.

CHAPTER TWO

Introduction to Infectious Disease

Man is host to a number of parasites. By convention the infectious diseases are regarded as those resulting from parasitism by small, often microscopic, forms of life—plant and animal. These infectious parasites include viruses, rickettsiae, bacteria, amoebae and fungi.

Again by convention parasitic diseases are sometimes distinguished from infections: the former are simply those in which the organism causing the disease is a larger one, like a worm, rather than smaller ones like bacteria, and this convention applies whether the worm is large and easily visible to the naked eye or where some stages are microscopic, as with microfilariae. Man also acts as a source of food to numerous blood-sucking arthropods—the vast 'joint-footed' class of the zoological classification, which not only includes the insects but also various bugs, fleas, lice, mites etc. Some of the arthropods are directly parasitic, attaching themselves to the body or body hair, and incapable of sustaining life for long away from the host. Whether leading an existence largely independent of man, like mosquitoes, or directly parasitic on him, like lice, these animals may be no more than an annoyance, causing an itch and perhaps superficial skin infections arising from scratching. Some of them, however, are carriers of disease, or, more technically, vectors of disease.

Vectors is the better word, so that 'carriers' may be reserved for those who carry an infection and can pass it on but are not affected by it themselves. Some vectors of infection are merely mechanical, simply transporting a pathogen in such a way as to infect a susceptible person. House flies, for instance, may carry amoebic dysentery from the exposed faeces of an infected person to the food about to be eaten by a susceptible one. Other vectors, in contrast, are essential to the development of the pathogen: thus some stages of the development of the malaria parasite take place within the body of the vector mosquito, while others take place within man (in some malarias within other animals, birds or mammals). There is a sense in which these mosquitoes and man are really alternate hosts to the parasite, but by convention the mosquitoes, and other arthropods essential to the life cycle of a particular parasite, are often referred to as disease vectors.

The pathogens of many infectious diseases act as stimuli to the protective mechanisms of the host's body, so that a varying degree of immunity may be conferred, and this may be more or less long-lasting. Some of the milder 'diseases' of childhood may be considered as simply the acquisition of the immunity to particular micro-organisms necessary to living in the communities necessary to man as a social animal. Most parents would agree that chickenpox, or varicella, comes in this category. German measles (rubella) might be placed there, and perhaps the more so in one sense, since the discovery in Australia that German measles in pregnant women is associated with an increased proportion of congenital defects in the babies born from the pregnancies affected by the virus, and it is better for females to acquire the immunity in childhood and avoid the risks during pregnancy in adult life.

Once experienced, these infectious diseases commonly confer long, perhaps lifelong, immunity on the host. Similarly, immunity to mumps can readily be seen as best acquired in childhood, since it seems to cause more severe illness in adults and to cause sterility in a small proportion of men victims. The virus moves from its normal focus in the parotid and other salivary glands through the lymphatic system to cause swelling in other glands, occasionally including permanent damage to the testes. Many parents would demur, however, at regarding measles or rubella, another virus infection, as a mere episode in the acquisition of desirable immunities, for it may cause severe illness, permanent damage to health in some children, and even some deaths, even in communities with high standards of medical care.

In a sense we have returned to the differing degrees of host-parasite adjustment from the biologist's viewpoint discussed earlier. Intuitively it seems that infections associated with little illness, with a high degree of host-parasite adjustment, may have attained this relatively stable relationship after a long period of living together with the host. The extreme case of host-parasite adjustment occurs in the commensal infections, like the harmless *Escherichia coli* already taken as an example, which share the host's meals from their ecological niche in the human gut. One can see a whole spectrum of differing degrees of host-parasite adjustment. But given the viewpoint of this book, it is better to explore this theme in relation to the community rather than to the individual, to think of immunity in the community rather than in the individual. Community immunity is important in relation to our next section.

Community immunity and endemic and epidemic diseases

Changing viewpoint slightly, then, the different degrees of host-parasite adjustment can be looked at from their effect on the community. High community immunity implies that most individuals in the community are wholly or partly immune to the infection. If they receive the infection, they are either not 'ill' at all, or their normal activities are only mildly inconvenienced by it; many of us are only slightly impeded in our daily activities by most infections by the cold virus. Infections are more commonly associated with a high degree of community immunity if the infection is endemic, ie constantly present in the population.

Take the case of measles, which may be considered as endemic even though the endemicity may take the form of periodic waves of the infection often referred to as epidemics. Endemicity taking this form is characteristically associated with relatively low community immunity to the infection. This is especially true of children, who have been born or lost any early immunity transmitted from their mother since the last 'epidemic' wave. Many are seriously indisposed, a few are very ill, and a small minority may even die directly or indirectly because of the infection. Most adults, on the other hand, have acquired immunity, often complete and lifelong, through infection in childhood. (We are leaving aside the possibility of mass immunization campaigns, though these are now feasible.)

Relatively low community immunity associated with 'epidemic' waves within a basically endemic pattern may be contrasted with the catastrophic epidemic, capable of causing severe illness and many deaths throughout the population at all ages in a community to which the particular infection is new, and where in consequence the community immunity is very low or absent. In the extreme case of true epidemic conditions a community may be decimated, or even almost wiped out. For example, measles had a devastating impact on several Pacific island populations in the nineteenth century, and even in the 1950s on Easter Island, on Greenland and the Faroes; and very sharp outbreaks occurred in nineteenth-century Australia at long intervals, during which a large population of susceptibles had time to build up.

To sum up, in an endemic area an infection may cause illness, chiefly among children, perhaps severe illness and some deaths; young babies may receive some congenital immunity from their mothers, but this commonly fades in childhood, the most susceptible period. The survivors of childhood enjoy a varying degree of immunity to the infection, so that in later years few people become seriously ill from the infection and fewer still die from it.

The pattern of disease is different under epidemic conditions. All age groups of the population are affected by more serious illness, perhaps with many deaths, depending on the disease, and particularly if any immunity conferred by the disease is relatively shortlived. The infection may still affect children somewhat more severely, for children born since the last epidemic will have little or no immunity to it; and there will be a large proportion of severe illness and deaths among old people. Think of a typical influenza epidemic in Britain! But, as compared with an endemic disease, there may be more serious demographic and economic effects on the middle age groups of the population—loss of wage-earning by breadwinners, and orphaning of dependent children if deaths are caused among parents. As we shall see in Chapter 4, malaria gives good examples of these contrasts between endemic and epidemic areas.

From the developed world I have chosen to deal with infectious hepatitis (the commonest form of jaundice), and influenza (Chapter 3). Infectious hepatitis is a debilitating and often long-lasting virus disease, important socially and economically as a drag on efficiency and family well-being. Influenza is discussed since it is still a major cause of illness and death even in the developed world, and the cause of the most recent of the really great and catastrophic pandemics, which occurred in the years following World War I.

From the underdeveloped world (Chapter 4) I discuss first malaria, the object of one of the great crusades to eradicate disease of the last 30 years, and still a major scourge of the tropical world, then two causes of blindness in the Third World, trachoma and river blindness or onchocerciasis.

CHAPTER THREE

Infectious Disease in the Developed World

Infectious hepatitis

This is a disease caused by a virus infection, and is a common though by no means the only cause of jaundice. It is primarily an intestinal disease, and commonly causes sickness and diarrhoea in its early stages; but much more fundamentally and more seriously it impairs the functioning of the liver, causing jaundice, nausea and lassitude, sometimes lasting many weeks. It causes serious loss of efficiency, not only to children attending school but also to many adults in their peak years of economic productivity and family responsibilities. It is transmitted, so far as is known at present, by direct carriage of the virus from person to person; this occurs, for example, by close personal contact, by ingestion from eating and drinking vessels contaminated by the saliva or faeces of infected persons, and by house flies acting as mechanical vectors. Polluted water, too, may sometimes be drunk or swallowed during swimming or bathing.

Infectious hepatitis normally causes much protracted and debilitating illness, rather than many deaths. Serum hepatitis is an exception: sometimes the infection reaches the bloodstream of a susceptible person through the blood of a person once affected, as in blood transfusions, occasional laboratory accidents or rarely on other occasions—blood from a scratch on a bramble coming from a leading runner in a hill-scrambling race has been known to enter the bloodstream of a later runner scratching himself on the same bramble.[1] Serum hepatitis at present seems to be a much more intractable problem than the more usual infection, causing much severe illness and a large proportion of deaths. A few hospitals of high repute have had sequences of cases of serum hepatitis, losing several skilled medical personnel as well as some patients.

The geography of infectious hepatitis

Infectious hepatitis may be endemic in underdeveloped countries, affecting many children but not adults, who have immunity. In these respects and in several aspects of its natural history it resembles the much more serious 'infantile paralysis' or 'acute anterior poliomyelitis' (or simply polio). The continual drain of hepatitis is a continual reminder of how much we owe in the prevention of polio to the work of Salk and others on prophylactic inoculations. Since the priority given to research on hepatitis has been much lower, only less effective immunization is available. An attack confers long-lasting, perhaps lifelong, immunity. In cool temperate countries there is a tendency for hepatitis to be a summer disease, perhaps because of greater activity by house flies, though heavier pollution of limited water supplies may play a part. In warm temperate countries, on Australian evidence, the disease does not have a clear seasonal incidence, and presumably this applies also to tropical countries.

Within developed countries the disease tends to have an epidemic cycle of about 5 years. It appears to have endemic foci, possibly in groups of immune carriers and more certainly taking this or other shape in large urban communities, for epidemic waves tend to spread from there. Since there will be a population of children without immunity, born since the last epidemic wave, there is some of the characteristic concentration of incidence in young children. Many adults have experienced a previous epidemic wave, but many are susceptible, too, and there is a good deal of adult illness. The spread of the infection can be followed in detail from some fascinating community case studies.

Thus Brownlea has studied a small township of 250 people in the northwest of New South Wales (Figure 8). He shows how the virus was brought in by a susceptible individual M6, a 6-year-old

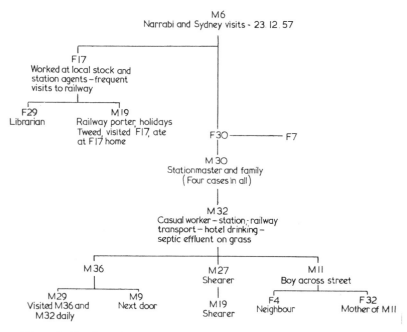

Figure 8. The flow of hepatitis virus between members of a small rural community in New South Wales. (Source: Brownlea, A. A., personal communication, 1964.)

boy who had made pre-Christmas visits to the large country town of Narrabri and also the state capital, Sydney; he became ill on 23 December 1957. He infected a 17-year-old girl stock dealer's clerk, a frequent visitor to the railway station (F17), and also his father (M30), a 30-year-old stationmaster. The boy's mother and sister also developed jaundice (F30 and F7). Then a 19-year-old porter, who was responsible for the disposal of sewage pails from the station, went down (M19), apparently as a result of visiting the girl (F17) and eating at her home. Both these young people had contact with the local librarian (F29) and one of them infected her. That particular lineage of hepatitis cases seems to have died out with this group.

The outbreak at the station, however, is thought to have infected a casual worker about local stock-rearing properties and the railway station, who went drinking at the local hotel, where septic tank effluent was discharged on to a grass field. You will see from the diagram that this part of the lineage or tree-diagram includes two further 'generations' of cases, numbering eight in all, and reflecting of course the close-knit community life in a small township. This is why it is comparatively easy to trace the movement of infectious hepatitis through such a community, as Dr W. N. Pickles of Wensleydale pointed out in his classic studies many years ago. Interpreting a very similar tree diagram of an epidemic of jaundice in Wensleydale in the 1920s, Dr Pickles began to suspect that the common link between the first victims must have been present at a village fête on 28 August:

After a prolonged search I found that a young girl who had begun with the disease on 23 August had been at the entertainment. I had actually seen her in bed in the morning and never dreamt she could have left it. She must have eluded me with great skill throughout the afternoon, since I was there myself and never set eyes on her. She spent the afternoon with E, another young girl, and was in the house of Mrs C, so that I think it is a fair presumption that she infected them and the other three. This young girl E, a maid in another village, infected four others. One was her employer's small son, another his friend, and another her own great-aunt. All this was reasonably clear. Of the fourth —M—there was some doubt. He was a rather pathetic little fellow of forty (since dead of tuberculous kidney) and denied all acquaintance with this young girl. However, his sister gave him away shamelessly. 'Robert not know Margaret?' said she, 'Why he's very fond of her—he generally goes in at the back door in the evenings and helps her to wash up.' Robert might well have said with Samson, 'If ye had not plowed with my heifer, ye had not found out my riddle'.[2]

The girl who wanted to go to the fête despite her jaundice caused at least thirteen other cases. More important for epidemiology, Pickles was able to confirm the incubation period of this disease, and establish it for other infections for the first time.

Such small-scale incidents can be aggregated, so that we can see broader epidemic wave patterns. We might expect modern transport movements to blanket whole tracts with the disease at a stroke. In fact the main epidemic wave rolls slowly across a country, as we can see from Figure 2, even though there are individual splashes of the disease far ahead of the wave crest and also behind the crest.

Both the broader and the local patterns have been studied by simulation methods. After a rather crude preliminary exercise by the writer, a much better simulation of a broad epidemic wave was devised by Chappell and Webber (Figure 9). An electronic network was used to simulate the towns and communications of New South Wales, and an electronic wave used to simulate the epidemic wave. The passage of the wave crest could be plotted by means of an oscilloscope, in which the wave appears like an animated graph on a television screen. This kind of 'hardware' model, as it is called, uses a grid of wires to simulate the trans-

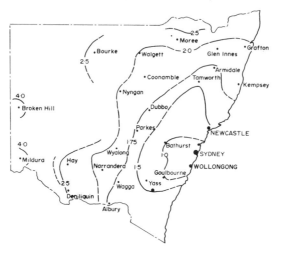

Figure 9. 'Map' showing outward movement of wave crest (of infectious hepatitis), by simple diffusion. 'Innovators' (carriers) are assumed to have increased at a uniform rate in Sydney, and to have meanwhile been diffusing steadily out into the state. At a certain level, increase in numbers ceased in Sydney (scaled to be 8 months after the process began); the 'map' shows the time, scaled in years, for maximum numbers to diffuse into each town in the model state. (Source: Chappell, J. M. A. and Webber M. J. 'Electrical Analogues of Spatial Diffusion Processes', *Regional Studies* 4, 1970, Fig 5, p 31.)

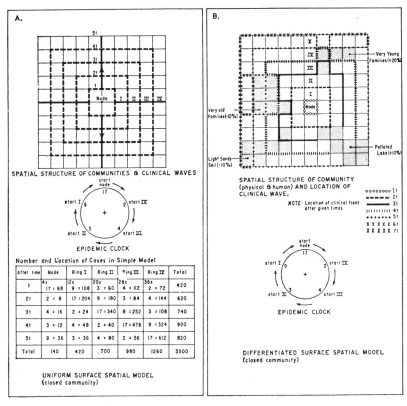

Figure 10. Modelling an infectious hepatitis epidemic. Model A represents random diffusion in successively wider zones I to IV, whereas in Model B the chances of successful spread by the virus have been modified in 'favourable' or 'unfavourable' populations. (Source: Brownlea, A. A. 'Modelling the Geographic Epidemiology of Infectious Hepatitis', in McGlashan, N. D. [ed]. *Medical geography: techniques and field studies*, Methuen/University Paperbacks, 1972, Fig 20.4, p 294.)

port movements between towns and cities, and is complementary to a rich literature on the mathematics of epidemics. This goes back at least as far as a paper by Sir Ronald Ross in 1916, and there is plenty of modern work in the field, which is called biomathematics.[3]

Given enough data about the variables present in the diffusion of the epidemic, a digital computer and an appropriate algebraic formula could be used to calculate and eventually to forecast the rate and pattern of the epidemic wave. A great deal of literature over the years has been devoted to epidemics in general; the principles are well understood but the data about the detailed behaviour of the epidemic are difficult to match up with the theory. Chappell and Webber, however, believe that the electronic wave or an analogue computer may be useful in the circumstances where so few of the variables can be given actual values that the computation from an algebraic formula cannot be done.

On the more local scale of Figure 10 Brownlea had complemented his ecological studies of the actual spread of the infection, as in Figure 2, by simulation studies. He assumes initially that there is random spread from a given source of infection, that is, from a given carrier or infected person the virus is spread randomly in successively larger zones, so that he could pass it on to someone moving in any direction. Qualifying this initially rather unreal assumption, Brownlea is able, for example, to allow for rather low spread into communities with a relatively stable and middle-aged to elderly population, which will tend to have a high community immunity. Low success rates for the virus are also envisaged by postulating housing on high ground or sandy soil, or main sewerage instead of septic tank or similar systems. Similarly he is able to allow for very high spread of the infection into an area, say, of very youthful population, with many children of low immunity, especially in housing areas on low ground, on heavy clays and near to the coastal lagoon where children may swim in polluted water (see Figure 10). These methods assist understanding. Potentially prediction based on similar approaches might be useful—for instance, in assessing priorities in campaigns to reduce the spread of infection or promote inoculation as that becomes more efficient and widely available.

Influenza

A virus infection, primarily of the air-passages, but with effects on the whole body such as fever, headache and weakness. The virus itself can be dangerous, but the special risk is added bacterial infection of the lungs. Of the estimated 20 million deaths in the pandemic (ie world-wide epidemic) of 1918–19, most were due to pneumonia to which the influenza made people highly vulnerable. Subsequent pandemics have been far less lethal.

An attack confers immunity to that strain of virus. Each successive wave of influenza, usually at intervals of some ten years, is due to a new strain of virus to which people are not immune. There are two explanations of the new strains, both probably valid. One is the evolution of modified forms of the virus; the other is infection of man by viruses that were previously confined to animals.

Effective vaccines can be prepared to give protection against known strains of influenza virus, but they will be useless against a new epidemic, when a new vaccine will be needed.[6]

It is almost impossible to write about influenza without mentioning the great pandemic of 1918–19, perhaps better dated 1918–21, to cover its spread across nearly the whole globe—as Peter Wingate does in that splendid passage from the *Penguin Medical Encyclopedia* above. Unprecedented in scale in modern times, it yet had antecedents. There was a major pandemic affecting many countries in 1889-94, with recurrences in 1895, 1900 and 1908. As often, the immediate cause of death was usually pneumonia, and it is worth noting that in Britain, for instance, influenza mortality in the 1900s was disproportionately high in the industrial towns, then subject to serious smoke pollution.

The 1918–21 pandemic was one of the most catastrophic of all epidemics, killing more than the millions who died on the several battlefronts of the 1914–18 war, and treating comparatively lightly only a few fortunate areas. The latter comprised, on the one hand, some lightly peopled lands far away from the main masses of population and movements of people, such as much of Australia; and, on the other hand, some tropical areas such as southern and eastern India where, despite high population densities, it seemed that conditions for transmission of a droplet infection were lacking, or, more likely, the virus lost virulence by a further mutation. Mapping of the distribution of influenza mortality in 1918–21 in a country like Britain, squarely on the path of the pandemic and at the end of an exhausting war, is not very rewarding, simply because the distribution patterns across the towns, villages and farms so closely reflect the distribution of population itself, among which the virus reaped a random harvest; it was not selective, say, of industrial towns, and was no respecter of privileged areas or groups. An outbreak of a virus disease in a military camp in the USA in 1976, which may have been caused by the spread of a zoonotic virus, swine fever, from pigs to men, has recently revived speculation that the 1918–21 pandemic may have been due to a massive attack on human populations, with little immunity, by the swine fever virus. However, this discussion will be based on the assumption of mutations in a human influenza virus rather than a zoonosis.

While the virus mutates, as the opening quotation notes, the mutation in a particular epidemic is often classed in relation to three main strains, labelled A, B and C: A is associated with widespread epidemics or pandemics, B with more localized epidemics, and C with sporadic cases or outbreaks. The pandemics cited above were attributed to the A strain, and the 'Asian flu' pandemic in the late 1950s was due to a fresh strain of the virus apparently mutating from the A strain and so classed as A2. Since it was a new strain, immunity to it was low all over the world, but fortunately it was generally less virulent than those of 1889 and 1918. It provides a good set of modern data, which have been analysed by geographers, and their findings will be outlined.[7]

The influenzal virus A2 appeared in early 1957. It caused an epidemic in south central China by February, reached Hong Kong by mid-April, and spread along routeways stretching from Hong Kong to many parts of the world. As with many epidemics and pandemics, the main epidemic wave crest was preceded by individual cases and sporadic outbreaks as noted in relation to infectious hepatitis earlier in this chapter, and sometimes referred to as pre-epidemic seeding.

Seeding was first caused by air travellers from the East, then by ships' crew and passengers (there still were passenger liners from the East!), and finally by people returning from the Continent, where they had met the advancing epidemic wave. Air travellers were as yet comparatively few, and their impact relatively small because they mainly lived in areas with low room densities, so that they were the less likely to pass on the virus. Some Pakistan Navy personnel flew into London on 13 June and were accommodated on a ship at Tilbury from which the virus spread. Infected ships' crews landed at Tilbury, Avonmouth, Sunderland, Jarrow and Manchester, and passengers at Southampton on 26 June. Liverpool received affected ships on 27 June and 1 July, and so on to a total of thirty-five ships carrying the virus by late October. Seeding increased as the main wave approached across Europe, reaching Britain by late August and then increasing as the schools' autumn term increased close contacts. The crest of the epidemic wave was reached in mid-October, reaching almost a million cases in a week, and it had virtually died down by late November.

We have already noted that mortality due directly to influenza does occur, but that many more deaths are due to bacterial infection of the lungs. Most of this comes through pneumonia caused by organisms such as *Pneumococcus* or *Diplococcus pneumoniae*, though mortality from bacterial pneumonia had been greatly reduced since the 1918–21 pandemic, by the use of antibiotics. Hunter and Young found that the 6,000 or so deaths attributable to the pandemic did not lend themselves to satisfactory statistical analysis, while incidence of influenza cases can only be calculated very broadly by indirect methods. They were particularly interested to map and analyse the spread of the pandemic through the crucial 12 weeks of the autumn of 1957, and in order to do this they were driven to base their calculations on cases of pneumonia (not deaths). Pneumonia is a notifiable disease, and its incidence is fairly accurately known. The next step was to compare the numbers of National Insurance sickness-benefit claims for influenza and for pneumonia over the period; this produced a figure of 417 cases of influenza to one case of pneumonia. The movement of the influenza virus across the country and the way it behaved in different communities were then studied, by means of the indirect evidence offered by the pneumonia notifications. The pneumonia notifications for a particular time or place were simply multiplied by 417 to produce an estimate of the influenza cases, and so the movement of the virus. (This is known as using a surrogate or simply substitute variable, and is quite a recognized method of analysis, provided the need to resort to this expedient is established and of course provided that the researchers put their cards on the table about what they are doing.)

Figure 13 shows the graph of the 1957 influenza epidemic in England and Wales, a component of the pandemic, as calculated from the pneumonia notifications. It shows a classic wave pattern very close to a theoretical prediction based on the numbers of cases and the period. There is one exception, that the base level of 'primary pneumonia' at the end of the epidemic is over twice that at the beginning; this is because the autumn normally sees a seasonal rise in respiratory disorders. In fact the very sharp peak superimposed on the normal gentle rise is an indication of low community immunity to the new strain of the virus.

Figure 11 shows the movement of the centre of gravity of the epidemic from the north-west of the Midlands towards the southeast, as it spread across the country, week by week. The unconventional but recognizable shape of England and Wales on

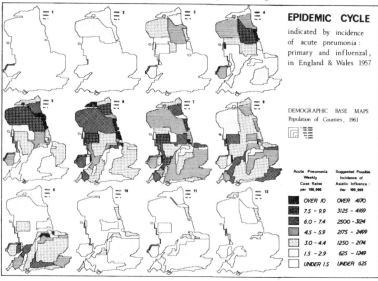

Figure 11. Influenza in England and Wales, 1957. The epidemic cycle is indicated by weekly rates. Maximum contrasts occur in weeks four and nine, heaviest and most widespread incidence in weeks six through to eight. (Source: Hunter, J. M. and Young, J. C. 'Diffusion of influenza in England and Wales', reproduced by permission from the *Annals of Assoc of Amer Geographers*, 61, 1971, Fig 5.)

49

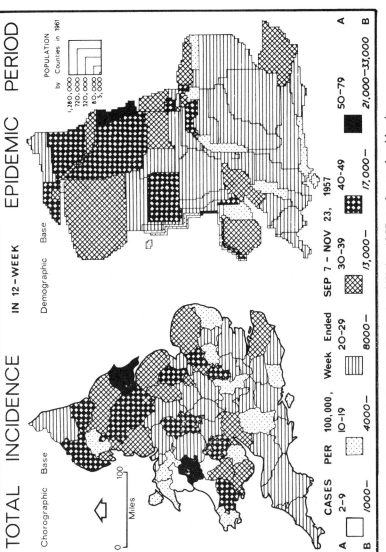

Figure 12. Influenza in England and Wales, 1957: twelve-week epidemic period, infection rates for (A) notification of acute pneumonia and (B) estimates of influenza based on the pneumonia rates (see text). (Source: as Figure 11, Hunter and Young, Fig 4.)

these maps is caused by their being drawn on a demographic base instead of an areal one; ie counties are drawn proportionally to county populations and not county areas. This method is discussed in the next paragraph in relation to Figure 12.

Figure 14 shows the movement of the epidemic in two different ways; the bottom diagram is easier to read for many people, but includes only five shadings for the nine weeks. Despite the early seeding in the London area, the epidemic began in the north, the epidemic wave there reaching its peak in early October, with 3–6 per cent of population falling sick in a week. Industrial South Wales and the West Midlands began a couple of weeks later, and 'peaked' a week after that. London and the South East began a week or two later again, and peaked in late October to early November. (Essex became a centre of dispersal in late September but soon peaked.) In mid-October the epidemic was almost countrywide. It retreated sooner from the north, and appeared to clear to the south like a weather depression moving from north-west to south-east. Let us turn to the total impact of the epidemic on different areas.

Figure 12 shows the then counties of England and Wales, shaded according to the incidence of pneumonia cases, in six classes, with relevant numerical values above the shadings (A); but the values can also be regarded as estimates of influenza incidence, using this particular surrogate as noted below the shadings (B). Here the left-hand map is drawn to scale to the familiar county areas and coastline of England and Wales, and for comparison the right-hand one on the demographic base. The latter map is less useful for comparing the influenza map with, say, a map of mean annual rainfall, but it does prevent the reader from overestimating the importance of sparsely peopled counties, such as Caernarvonshire in North Wales, or underestimating the impact of populous counties like the West Riding of Yorkshire. The estimates suggest that 11·5 per cent of the total population were affected by influenza, rising to 20 per cent or so in much of northern England, the East and West Midlands, the head of the Severn estuary, and central and South Wales. The main groups of low rates (individual counties' rates should not be regarded as necessarily of significance) are in north and west Wales and in

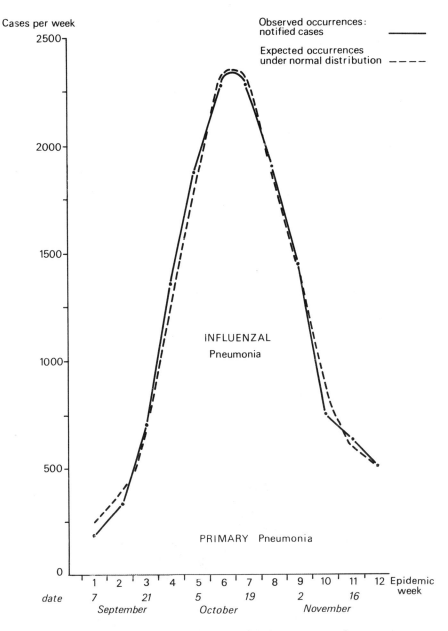

Figure 13. Graph of influenzal pneumonia and primary pneumonia September–November, 1957. (Source: as for Figure 11, Hunter and Young, Fig 2.)

four counties spread between Greater London and the Midlands. There appears to be some relation with the large industrialized towns, and Hunter and Young draw attention to a family resemblance between their map and G. M. Howe's map of bronchitis mortality (Figures 50 and 51).

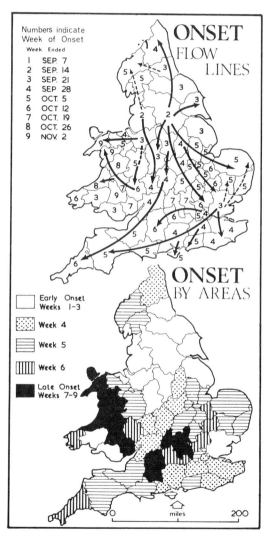

Figure 14 Influenza in England and Wales, 1957: virus flow lines shown by weeks of epidemic onset (Source: as Figure 11, Hunter and Young, Fig 7.)

Hunter and Young have mapped and analysed both the total incidence of influenza and the inferred movements of the virus in the area between the Mersey and Humber (Figures 11 and 14). Early coastal foci included the major seaports of Liverpool and Hull, and also Middlesbrough, but there were also inland foci, in manufacturing towns and cities. Onset of the epidemic was delayed in rural areas, but these were heavily affected later. An important finding from these studies was that cities with large textile mills whose workers included immigrants with contacts with the East experienced early infection, followed by a rapid spread and an early peak, mainly among factory workers, with a slower upsurge of infection in the populace, causing a second peak peculiar to cities with large closed populations of this type.

The epidemic did not necessarily spread steadily outward from this initially important northern focus. Hunter and Young show how it spread north to Newcastle; then, as it were against the main northward current, the epidemic wave moved southward into County Durham, leaving industrial Tees-side lightly affected. Finally Hunter and Young compared the distribution pattern of influenza, as estimated, with what might be expected by comparison with 'population potential' (an analogy with gravity), which is a way of allowing for the total impact of population not only in numbers but also by their proximity to or distance from other population groups. Hunter and Young show that population potential could have been used early in the epidemic to forecast the severely affected areas and, less obviously, the pathway from north-west to south-east (along a ridge of high potential). High room densities were a better index of rapid spread of the virus than population density as such.

A much greater anomaly than the low incidence in Tees-side already noted was that Greater London, with early seeding and a massive population of which substantial parts live at high room densities, was comparatively lightly affected by the epidemic. Perhaps the areas of overcrowding there were offset by the very large prosperous areas with low room densities.

This study of influenza, like some of the geographical work on infectious hepatitis, shows some potential for prediction and practical use ahead of an epidemic wave.

CHAPTER FOUR

Infectious Disease in the Underdeveloped World

In the underdeveloped world infectious diseases (used broadly to include the parasitic diseases) are proportionately much more important than in the developed world. Often they are insect-borne, or arthropod-borne (to use the broader terms for the zoologists' 'joint-footed' order, including not only the insects but also spiders, mites etc). Many of these infections are popularly taken as 'tropical diseases', but in fact several are or have been of considerable importance in the temperate countries in the developed world. Yellow fever has caused sharp epidemics as far north as Bristol and Halifax, Nova Scotia. Malaria caused much of the debility and killing 'agues' of the marshes and fens of lowland England and the Netherlands. Cholera caused catastrophic epidemics over much of Britain during the mid-nineteenth century. Plague of course swept across all Europe as the Black Death in the fourteenth century and decimated London in 1665. Leprosy was formerly endemic in much of Europe, with King Robert the Bruce as a celebrated victim—one can hardly think of him as a patient—and it survives as a small but significant public-health problem in such temperate countries as Iceland and Norway, and even in Australia, though that is one-third tropical.

The retreat of these diseases from temperate areas was due, more often than not, to economic development and changes in standards of living rather than to any specific measures taken against them. We may well think that this is a matter of profound significance, yet it is by no means easy to follow through the chain of events, disease by disease, which caused the change. Malaria is thought to have retreated from England primarily because improvements in agriculture and housing in the nineteenth century separated human dwellings from cattle sheds. The main vector of the alluvial valleys was *Anopheles messeae*, and in the salt marshes *A. atroparvus*, both of which preferred to suck blood from cattle than from humans, and remained round cattle sheds rather than houses after the separation took place. Vector mosquitoes are still common in Britain, and, given a source of infection in the blood of an infected person, usually one recently returned from the tropics, can transmit malaria. This occurred on a considerable scale in the Thames marshes after World War I and to a much smaller extent after World War II. Transmission in London in the early 1950s was traced to *Anopheles plumbeus*, which bred in tiny pools of rainwater held in rot holes in the crutches of plane trees in London squares.

We are often reminded that cholera can still spread to Britain, probably the more readily in summer, in these days of rapid air transport of immigrants from South Asia and holidaymakers returning from some Mediterranean resorts. It is usually quickly suppressed by isolation and immunization of contacts. But the main retreat of cholera in the nineteenth century probably owed more to general improvements in water supplies, housing and

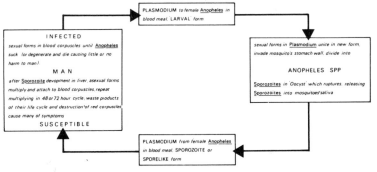

Figure 15. The malaria cycle, a simple flow diagram.
(Source: Learmonth, A. T. A.)

environmental hygiene generally than to specific health measures. Rather similarly, improvements in domestic and personal cleanliness are probably responsible in the main for the retreat of plague as a widespread and serious public-health problem in the developed world. Sporadic cases may occur, however, and there are, for instance, a few cases in most years in the USA round the enzootic area in the arid and semi-arid south-west.

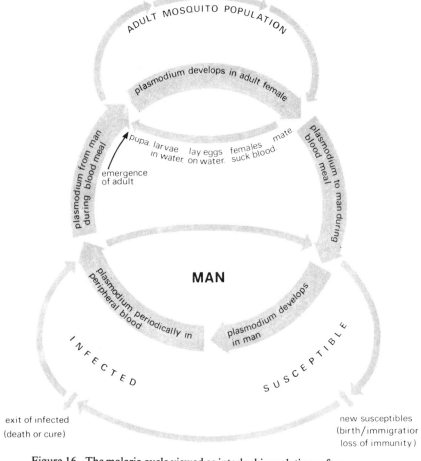

Figure 16. The malaria cycle viewed as interlocking relations of man, mosquito and malaria parasite. (Source: Open University. 'The population explosion, an interdisciplinary approach', in *Understanding Society* course, Fig 33.6, p 45.)

Malaria

The malaria cycle

Malaria has already been referred to several times, on the assumption that of all the arthropod-borne diseases the cycle is best known to the man in the street. However, Figure 15 shows some of the main elements of the cycle diagrammatically, and the reader will see that *Anopheles* mosquitoes are indeed alternate hosts of the protozoal parasite, as noted earlier, rather than merely mechanical vectors; both man and mosquito are essential to the maintenance of the cycle, on present knowledge, so far as the main species of *Plasmodium* parasitic on man are concerned. (Infection of man by monkey malaria under 'natural' as against laboratory conditions, however, was proved more than once several years ago; and birds, rodents and other animals are also known to have their own malaria cycles.) Figure 16 is a complementary representation of the malaria cycle in man that places more emphasis on how the mosquitoes' life cycle fits in with the circulation of *Plasmodium* between man and mosquito. The complex movements and manifold activities of man that affect man–mosquito contacts have not, of course, been even hinted at in this diagram.

The main species of Plasmodium *affecting man, and their changing geography*

Figure 17 shows the distribution over the globe of the main species of *Plasmodium* affecting man as it was about 1950. *P. falciparum*, which causes the classical malignant tertian or sub-tertian fever (the fever recurring about every 48 hours), is shown as very widespread in the tropics, especially in Africa and the Americas.

P. vivax, causing the classical benign tertian fever, covered the same areas but was dominant in much of Asia and extended into temperate latitudes.

P. malariae, causing quartan fever, ie about every 72 hours, was locally important but usually subsidiary to *P. falciparum* and *P. vivax*.

P. ovale, generally causing a comparatively mild and short

58

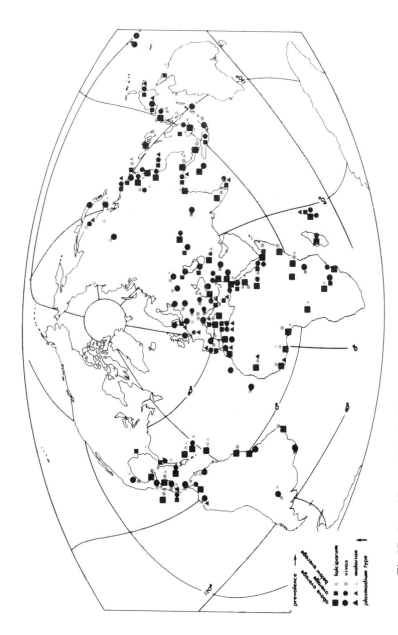

Fig 17. A world map of the distribution of the main parasites of human malaria, c1950. (Source: May, J. M. 'World atlas of diseases No. 3. World distribution of malaria vectors, *Georg Rev*, 41.)

illness, occurred mainly in the forested lowlands of West Africa and parts of East Africa.

These patterns have changed, largely because of the malaria control campaigns. *P. vivax* now has much the same distribution as *P. falciparum* had in 1950, having been banished from many temperate and even tropical summer rainfall areas like India (though with occasional recrudescence, as several times in Sri Lanka and quite severely in India from 1966 onwards). *P. falciparum* has tended to retreat, especially in the tropical Americas, though it remains in some drug-resistant areas and has formed a significant part of the resurgence of malaria in a belt across middle India.

P. malariae has a very long life in the human host, and so has managed to linger on even in areas of good malaria control, such as Rumania, and perhaps to become proportionately more important in the tropics. *P. ovale* seems little affected by the eradication campaigns, but has been reported from New Guinea and the Philippines. Its forest ecology suggests that it may prove to be a zoonosis, an animal disease into which man blunders, as it were, like yellow fever. *P. malariae*, again, has been found in chimpanzees in West Africa; but it must be stressed that the transmission from monkeys to man referred to earlier is by another species of the parasite not commonly found in man—*P. knowlesi.*

The evolution of the complex interlocking cycles that come together as the malaria cycle of our diagrams is a controversial topic, and naturally evidence is very difficult to gather. It has been suggested that *Plasmodium* has evolved from intestinal protozoa, among which close relatives have been identified, and that the genus became specialized into alternate parasitism on animals and on mosquitoes by evolution to fill a vacant ecological niche, as it were.[1]

It has already been noted that infectious diseases often affect a community differently if they occur in epidemic rather than endemic form, the epidemic tending to cause severe illness throughout the age groups, and the endemic severe illness and deaths in children, milder illness in adults and perhaps more severe cases and mortality among the old. In relation to malaria this phenomenon was observed by Sir Rickard Christophers in the 1920s in an iron-mining camp in Singhbhum in north-eastern peninsular India, when he noticed that locally recruited tribal people were comparatively immune to the prevalent *vivax* malaria, but that Bengali clerical staff brought in by the mining companies went down with severe attacks. Since then a great deal of attention has been paid to the spectrum of host-parasite relations from epidemic to endemic, and the World Health Organisation has classified endemicity by means of the simple though by no means certain indicator of enlarged spleens in children along the following lines:

1 Hypo-endemic   —childhood spleen rate below 10 per cent (children of 2–10 years)
2 Meso-endemic   —10–24 per cent
3 Highly endemic   —25–49 per cent
4 Hyper-endemic   —50–74 per cent
5 Holo-endemic   —75 per cent and over
6 Super-endemic   —75 per cent and over, associated with almost complete freedom from adult illness and low adult spleen rates maintained over long periods.

Though superseded by laboratory examination of blood specimens, the spectrum of degrees of endemicity remains valid, though altered in many parts of the world by control campaigns. Categories 1 and 2, together with areas without any indication of malaria, are naturally those where epidemic malaria might sweep through all ages, causing much severe illness and perhaps many deaths, while the higher numbers grade towards the case with late infant and child illness and mortality succeeded by comparative immunity in adults, which becomes substantial as noted under category 6 under the term super-endemicity. So far as is known, perfect host-parasite adjustment where adult illnesses are entirely lacking does not occur in human malaria. It may occur in isolated communities where there has been a long period of co-existence by man, *Plasmodium* and *Anopheles*, but such isolated and undisturbed communities can be few in number nowadays, and if they were known and studied they would not be undisturbed.

The malarial mosquito

Anopheline mosquitoes are widespread throughout the world

except for the cold deserts and much of the hot deserts. Different species seem to vary in 'efficiency' as vectors or alternate hosts—some species may simply prefer other prey, birds or rodents perhaps—but malaria does have the potential to be a world-wide disease, and indeed has approached that status at times in the past. However, there is a paradox here. In a sense malaria is a local disease, despite its world potential, because there are many species of *Anopheles* and these tend to have particular ecological preferences. Some have adapted to live close to or in houses or cattle sheds much of the time, resting there in shady spots during hot days or in cosy places on cold nights. Some have particular biting times—at dusk or dawn or in the middle of the night. The gravid adult female mosquito has particular preferences for breeding places, shown in her mating dance and also very significantly in her choice of a particular sort of water surface upon which to lay her eggs, where they will hatch and spend their early life as larvae (or 'wrigglers') and pupate before emerging as adults. The water is usually still but must not be stagnant or heavily polluted for this genus of mosquitoes, though other disease vectors do breed in organically polluted water, and certain species in running streams.

One must remember, however, that such ecological preferences are not necessarily fixed and immutable, nor absolutely consistent throughout a particular species of *Anopheles*. For instance, *A. stephensi* in Bombay became adapted to urban life, in house water cisterns and the like, and may even have evolved strains particularly suited to closely urban habitat—after all, mosquito generations succeed each other quickly! This vector is shown as having extended its territory in the latest maps of the National Institute of Communicable Diseases in New Delhi, as compared with that shown in Figure 18. Again, the malaria control campaigns have shown that some strains of a widespread African forest and temporary pool breeder like *A. gambiae* might be wiped out by residual (long-lasting) insecticides like DDT, but that if spraying stops, other 'wilder' strains emerge from the rain forest to occupy the 'ecological vacuum'.

Very importantly, the flight range of many important vector species is fairly small, often about half a mile, though some West

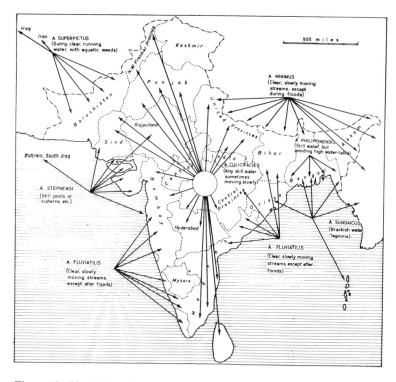

Figure 18. The Indian sub-continent, main malaria vectors c1945. The modern map has additional sites of *Anopheles stephensi* in south-eastern India and additional vectors in north-eastern India. (Source: Covell in Learmonth, A. T. A. 'Some contrasts in the regional geography of malaria in India and Pakistan', *Trans of Inst of British Geographers*, 23, 1957, Fig 2, p 39.)

African species have been proved to fly for several miles and even short-range species may be carried for several miles by strong winds. Even so, it is this combination of local dominance by particular species, with particular ecological preferences and limited flight range, which accounts for the local nature of malaria.

The way in which local patterns mount up into broader patterns may be illustrated from Figures 19 to 21. Figure 18 comes from a publication by a director of the Malarial Survey of India just before the launching of the great control campaigns, upon which I have given the barest indication of the breeding preferences of the different species. Figure 19 is a classic map of endemic (and humid) areas and of epidemic (and arid and semi-

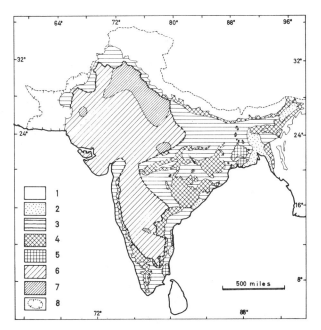

Figure 19. Malaria, Indian regional patterns.
1 Areas of 5,000ft (non-malarious).
2 Known healthy plains (spleen rates less than 10 per cent). Now somewhat
  smaller area in East Bengal than shown on map.
3 Moderate to high endemicity of more or less static character, the intensity
  depending on local surroundings; seasonal variation moderate, fulminant
  epidemics unknown.
4 Hyper-endemicity of hilly jungle tracts and *terai* land.
5 Probably hyper-endemic hill areas.
6 Hyper-endemicity other than hill areas.
7 Variable endemicity associated with dry tracts, usually showing
  autumnal rise in fever incidence (potential epidemic areas), spleen rate low
  except for years following epidemics, or in special local circumstances,
  and much affected by conditions of irrigation.
8 Known areas liable to fulminant epidemicity (diluvial) malaria. Spleen
  rate dependent on occurrence of epidemics, high during and immediately
  after such, slowly falling to low rates in course of half a decade or so.
9 Unsurveyed.
  The heavy pecked line marks the broad division between the endemic and
  epidemic regions of India and Pakistan. (Source: see Figure 20.
  Christophers, S. R. and Sinton, J. A. in Learmonth, 1957, Fig 1, p 38.)

arid) tracts bearing a family resemblance to the spread of cases
during the resurgence of 5–6 million in 1975. Figures 20 and 21
show typical breeding places, the former of the main vector of the

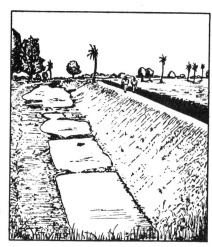

Figure 20. Breeding place of malaria vector *Anopheles culicificacies*. (Source: as Figure 18, Learmonth, 1957, Fig 5, p 43.)

whole sub-continent, *A. culicifacies*, and the latter of a very efficient vector of forest and tea-garden environments, *A. minimus*, which breeds in clear flowing streams except during floods, when the gravid female lays her eggs in temporary pools. When I presented a paper at a conference in the mid-1950s containing these and other illustrations of the links between anopheline ecology and the geography of malaria, it was criticized as being of merely historical rather than current interest, since malaria was well on the way to eradication. Yet the sharp recrudescence of malaria in India today has been sufficient to justify renewed interest in the topic.

Despite this setback, malaria control in India has been one of the great success stories of recent times. This was partly because the country could command good organization and a sufficiently well educated and diligent staff to carry out a campaign of house-spraying, and partly because the main vector species were house-haunting, so that house-spraying was effective; and house-spraying does not demand a great deal of active cooperation from masses of people. A particularly significant point, especially in view of the recent resurgence of the disease, is that near-eradication was achieved so that spraying was more or less stopped some years ago—partly to guard against the considerable danger that vector mosquitoes might develop immunity to the insecticides. This implies that renewed spraying has a good chance of success, assuming that the mosquitoes retain their house-haunting character. The interlocking cycles of Figure 16 may be thought of as broken by attacking mainly the adult mosquito phase at the top of the diagram, and this is true of much of the seasonal malarial territory of the world in which malaria control or eradication has been achieved since the end of World War II. We might contrast this with the retreat of malaria from England, where the cycle was broken by improvement in housing and stock-farming technology. Sometimes a combination of techniques may be necessary, perhaps house-spraying against adult mosquitoes combined with spraying bodies of water to kill larvae, or house-spraying combined with treatment of the people with drugs—particularly if the particular *Plasmodium* is likely to be reduced to such a low level that spraying can be stopped. Figure 22 illustrates such a combination of techniques from Morocco.

In contrast is Figure 23, from the equatorial rain-forest tract of Cameroon: here there is indeed a combination of house-spraying and treatment of the people with drugs, though both are regarded as only partially successful. In a hyper-endemic area several species of *Plasmodium* may well be present, and regular drug dosing would demand the co-operation of all the people in a degree much greater than that needed for house-spraying; thus it is easy to visualize that mass campaigns using therapeutic or pre-

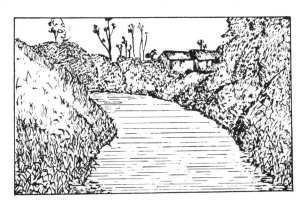

Figure 21. Breeding place of malaria vector *Anopheles minimus*. (Source: as Figure 18, Learmonth, 1957, Fig 17, p 54.)

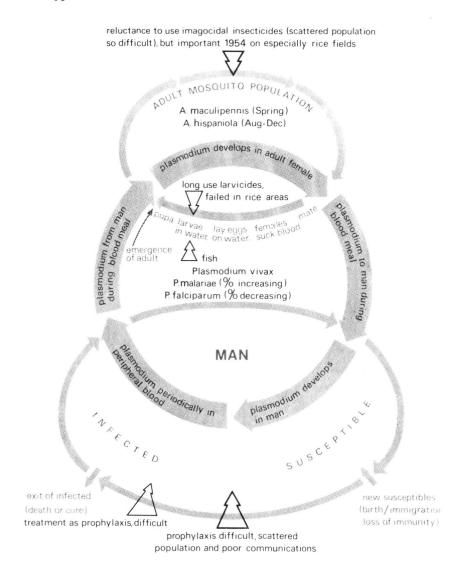

reluctance to use imagocidal insecticides (scattered population so difficult), but important 1954 on especially rice fields

ADULT MOSQUITO POPULATION

A. maculipennis (Spring)
A. hispaniola (Aug-Dec)

plasmodium develops in adult female

long use larvicides,
failed in rice areas

plasmodium from man during blood meal

pupa larvae lay eggs females mate in water on water suck blood

emergence of adult

fish

Plasmodium vivax
P. malariae (% increasing)
P. falciparum (% decreasing)

plasmodium to man during blood meal

MAN

plasmodium periodically in peripheral blood

plasmodium develops in man

INFECTED

SUSCEPTIBLE

exit of infected
(death or cure)
treatment as prophylaxis, difficult

prophylaxis difficult, scattered
population and poor communications

new susceptibles
(birth/immigration
loss of immunity)

Figure 22. Breaking the malaria cycle—Morocco. (Source: Learmonth, A. T. A. in Howe, G. M. [ed]. *World Medical Geography*, Academic Press, Fig 12.)

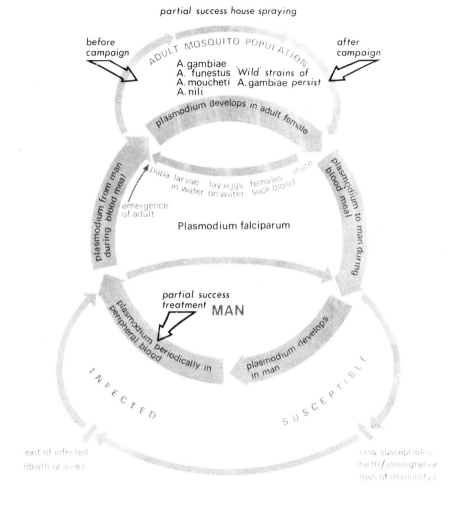

Figure 23. Attempting to break the malaria cycle—Cameroon. (Source: as Figure 22, Learmonth, Fig 8.)

ventive drugs might have limited success. On the other hand, measures against the mosquito have also had limited success, and in particular the persistence of 'wild' strains of *Anopheles gambiae* is noted on the diagram.

A. funestus in Africa is the classical vector breeding in permanent bodies of water, and with this comparatively restricted range, campaigns against it have been relatively successful. On the other hand, *A. gambiae* in Africa has always been a successful breeder in all sorts of bodies of water, many of them temporary—from pools of rainwater in discarded food cans to elephants' foot-prints. Breeding places, therefore, are myriad and ever-changing, so that anti-larval campaigns cannot well be contemplated. Moreover, even if strains comparatively closely adapted to human settlements are wiped out there are the so-called 'wild' strains noted on Figure 23; these do not use houses as resting places, but seek refuge in the forest, where spraying cannot be done. Such 'wild' strains commonly emerge from the forests to occupy the vacant niche left by more 'domesticated' strains that have succumbed to house-spraying.

In an environment much more susceptible to all-out attack upon *Anopheles*, in Sardinia, eradication of all known vector species was attempted some years ago; despite much more seasonal variation (the hot dry Mediterranean summer does not favour anopheline breeding), and comparatively restricted breeding sites in much less rainy terrain, it was found that, after spraying ceased, vector mosquitoes returned to many former breeding places. Even if the particular species was not the same as before the campaign, the newly vacant ecological niches were filled by other vector species. If this is true of Sardinia, in conditions comparatively hostile, or at least where the cycle is comparatively fragile and easily broken, how much more difficult is it in Cameroon or the rain forests of Zaire!

It is for this reason that the world crusade of malaria eradication has been modified in the areas of perennial mosquito-breeding and myriad breeding places towards malaria control, gradually extending in area—and therefore taking advantage of the fact that malaria is in a sense a local phenomenon, as noted earlier. In fact many of the workers closest to the problem believe that ultimately the malarial cycle can best be broken under these conditions by all-round economic development. This is probably true even if current work on a vaccine against malaria should prove successful. If so, malaria will retreat, along with many other adverse features of community health, such as high infant and child mortality.

The nature of the malaria cycle is such that almost from the time of its discovery much field research, as distinct from laboratory or clinical work, has been of an essentially geographical character. The writer has reviewed some very stimulating work by medical men.[2] Geographers have been able to offer some contributions in recent years. For example, a malaria control project in northern Nigeria met unexpected difficulties owing to the seasonal migration of thousands of people from controlled to uncontrolled and malarious areas, reactivating the cycle on their return; and the malariologist was able to call on a human geographer who had studied these migratory movements to advise on possible courses of action there and later in other parts of Africa and south-western Asia.[3]

One geographer, Ann Coles, contributed a great deal towards basic malaria survey work in the former Trucial States in the Arabian peninsula, lending field and cartographic skills and critical interpretation of data in poorly mapped or untapped terrain.[4] Geographical analysis can claim to offer fresh insights on occasions. For instance, the malaria cycle in Trinidad is unique in that a chief vector, *Anopheles bellator*, breeds in the small quantities of rainwater trapped at the base of epiphytes (bromeliads) growing on rain-forest trees, though not directly parasitic on them; this brings about particular relations with cocoa plantations, whose two-storey houses have their upper floors roughly at the mosquitoes' level. Study of the historical geography shows the interplay of this vector with the coastal brackish-water and rice-paddy species *A. aquasalis*, with different land-use patterns, genetic elements in the population and control measures.[5]

In conclusion, a pedagogic model rather than a research model of a hypothetical malarial continent is set out in Figures 24–35 in the hope that they will provide some sort of synthesis.

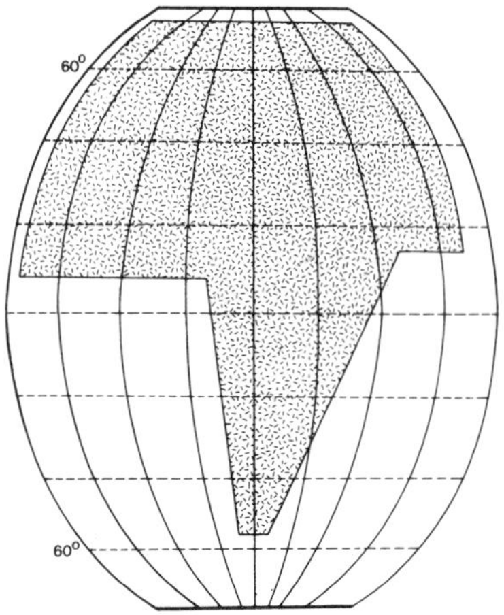

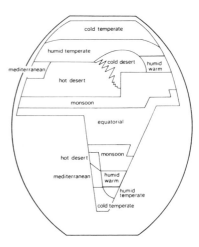

Figure 24. A 'model' of a hypothetical malarial continent, initial stage, simple and massive. (Source: as Figure 22, Learmonth, Fig 5.1.)

Figure 25. The main climatic zones of the continent. (Source: as Figure 22, Learmonth, Fig 5.2.)

Figure 24 represents the hypothetical continent as first envisaged—simple, massive, and stretching from about 75°N to some 55°S, where it simulates the narrower southern peninsulas of the real continents. Assumptions, some at least gradually removed in the later stages of the model, include low to undulating relief; bodies of water in various forms (still, running etc) used by different species of *Anopheles* for breeding; a uniform distribution of human population and of *Plasmodium*, both of density enough to sustain the malaria cycle; and universal 'underdevelopment', so that the cycle is not inhibited by human technology.

Figure 25 represents the main climatic zones, while Figure 26 brutally simplifies the implications of the climates for anopheline breeding, taking only the conditions of the warmest and coolest months as providing or not providing (a) suitable temperatures and (b) suitable bodies of water for *Anopheles* to breed. (Tem-

			Winter	Summer
1	cold temperate	temperature	O	O
		water	w	w
2	humid temperate	temperature	O	T
		water	w	w
3	cold desert	temperature	O	T
		water	o	o
4	mediterranean	temperature	T	T
		water	w	o
5	hot desert	temperature	T	T
		water	o	o
6	monsoon	temperature	T	T
		water	o	w
7	humid warm	temperature	T	T
		water	w	w
8	equatorial	temperature	T	T
		water	w	w

Figure 26. Table of influence of warmest and coldest months and of rainfall conditions on Anopheline activity in each climatic zone. (Source: as Figure 22, Learmonth, Fig 5.3.)

peratures roughly over 16°C with average relative humidities about 60 per cent are treated as favourable, temperatures over 35°C with relative humidities under 25 per cent as unfavourable; these are for purposes of the model rather than for serious specialized analysis of mosquito environments.) Figure 27 links these relations with malarial conditions, and illustrates the socio-economic and demographic impacts of endemic and epidemic conditions argued earlier.

In Figure 28 the model is modified, in order to begin the removal of some simplifying assumptions. (For the writer one function of a model is manipulation, to see if the process can add to understanding of a problem.) The continent receives new features: a mediterranean-type sea; mountain arcs of Alpine-Himalayan type; a plateau comparable to those of East Africa or Brazil; and a delta analogous to those of Rhine, Nile, Niger and Ganga-Brahmaputra or perhaps Mekong. Figure 29 carries on with the implications for malaria distribution of the changes, with malarious hot deltas etc.

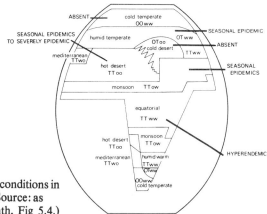

Figure 27. Malarial conditions in the climatic zones. (Source: as Figure 22, Learmonth, Fig 5.4.)

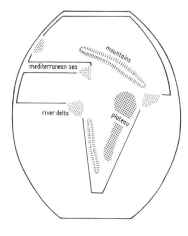

Figure 28. The continent modified to include a 'mediterranean' sea, mountain arcs, plateaux, and deltas. (Source: as Figure 22, Learmonth, Fig 5.5.)

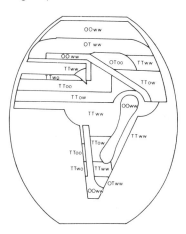

Figure 29. The effects of changes in the continent on malarial zones. (Source: as Figure 22, Learmonth, Fig 5.6.)

Figures 30–5 represent manipulations of the model to represent the impact of malaria eradication in different zones. Figure 30 shows a western European type of malarial retreat through improvements in agricultural and housing technology; and Figure 31 shows the impact of campaigns with DDT etc against adult *Anopheles*, locally complemented by the use of anti-larval measures and the use of mass therapy or prophylaxis. Note that both Figures 30 and 31 show locally resistent foci of malaria, while Figure 32 indicates local areas of control in rain-forest climates and perennial breeding in myriad bodies of water, innumerable anopheline retreats and resting places, and 'wild' strains like those of *A. gambiae* noted from Cameroon. Finally Figure 33 summarizes the picture of this group.

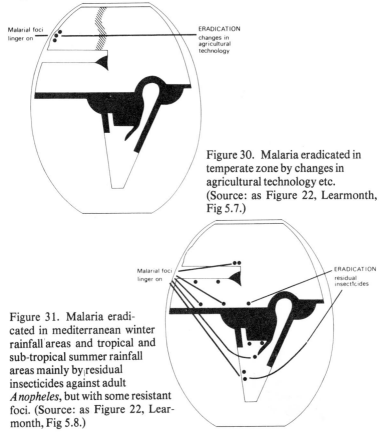

Malarial foci linger on

ERADICATION changes in agricultural technology

Figure 30. Malaria eradicated in temperate zone by changes in agricultural technology etc. (Source: as Figure 22, Learmonth, Fig 5.7.)

Malarial foci linger on

ERADICATION residual insecticides

Figure 31. Malaria eradicated in mediterranean winter rainfall areas and tropical and sub-tropical summer rainfall areas mainly by residual insecticides against adult *Anopheles*, but with some resistant foci. (Source: as Figure 22, Learmonth, Fig 5.8.)

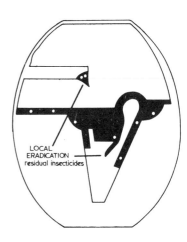

Figure 32. Malaria resistant in main zone of perennial malaria, but with eradication in local areas. (Source: as Figure 22, Learmonth, Fig 5.9.)

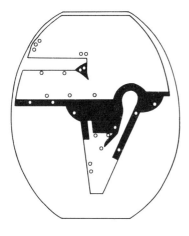

Figure 33. Summary map of effects of malaria control. (Source: as Figure 22, Learmonth, Fig 5.10.)

Figure 34. Effects on malaria control of human migration across border between controlled and uncontrolled areas. (Source: as Figure 22, Learmonth, Fig 5.11.)

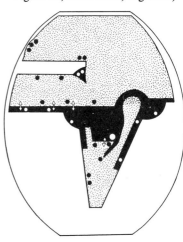

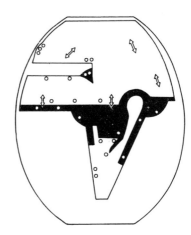

Figure 35. Effects on malaria
control of movement of climatic
belts. (Source: as Figure 22, Learmonth, Fig 5.12.)

The last two versions of the model represent further manipulations. Figure 34 sketches the effect of such migrations and
nomadism as the population movements studied by Prothero.
Figure 35 reminds us that climatic belts can move to and fro: that
a Bombay year can invade the Punjab, as in 1912, causing a
catastrophic epidemic; and that a Deccan dry plateau year can
invade the Wet Zone of Sri Lanka (Ceylon), as in 1935, bringing a
very severe epidemic caused by Dry Zone *Anopheles* and the very
lethal *falciparum* malaria.

Two causes of blindness: trachoma and onchocerciasis

Blindness is but the tip of the iceberg of eye disease, but such a
severe disability, combined with comparatively reliable data,
justifies its inclusion in a work of this kind. Blind people, like
coloured immigrants in a white population, are easily identifiable,
and the economic and social consequences of blindness are so
serious that for this reason also the blind stand out in the health
records of many countries, even if the general quality of statistics
is not good.

There are marked geographical differences in incidence and
type of blindness. The reader will not be surprised to know that
the developing countries have more than their share of both eye
disease and blindness; this is entirely in line with the state of
underdevelopment—with the vicious circle of poverty, poor living
conditions, poor nutrition, poor hygiene and lack of opportunity

to raise living standards. It is in line too with the retreat of many of the identical eye diseases from now developed countries without specific campaigns against them but simply as part of the process of development and raising of living standards.

To put the two case studies selected for this chapter in broader perspective, trachoma is an infectious disease of the eye affecting some 500,000,000 people in the world, and responsible for some 6,000,000 cases of blindness; and Northern Ghana, where one of our studies of river blindness was made, has an incidence of blindness some fifteen times as great as the rate in Europe—1 blind person per 33 people, as compared with 1 in 500 in Europe—and almost half of these are caused by 'river blindness' or onchocerciasis. Professor Ida Mann expresses the difference between Africa and Europe, the USA or Australia in almost epigrammatic form: 'Just as we could generalize about the African picture with *infection, blindness and malnutrition* so we can say of our own ophthalmic landscape that it is characterized by *cultural, industrial, genetic, iatrogenic and geriatric disease*'.[6]

Iatrogenic disease, not necessarily related to eyes, is disease associated with medicine or physicians, and geriatric disease with old age. The former arises mainly as side-effects of drugs, from quinine (for malaria) or emetine (for dysentery) to salicylates in aspirin, some skin salves or some of the commonly used tranquillizers. Geriatric eye disease includes glaucoma, which is caused by high pressure within the eye, and cataract or opacity of the lens of the eye; obviously geriatric diseases, like many diseases of middle and old age, increase in importance with increased expectation of life.

Cultural eye disease would cover cases associated with fireworks at Guy Fawkes' day bonfires, cosmetics, rash observations of an eclipse of the sun, or sunbathing, sailing or fishing into the sun, and many other cases. Industrial cases arise in both town and country, the more so if, as in Australia, a 'he-man' tradition operates against the regular use of protective goggles etc against flying sparks or splinters, and wherever agriculture is highly mechanized.

Genetic diseases include *Ophthalmia neonatorum*, often though not always caused by gonorrhoea and usually curable by antibiotics nowadays; congenital cataract and glaucoma; and the small proportion of congenital deformities of the eyes or optic nerves, including *Retinitis pigmentosa*, an overdevelopment of the connective tissue of the retina at the expense of the nerve elements. Some congenital defects are due to syphilis.

In the developing countries, in contrast, the emphasis is on infectious diseases and on those affecting young to middle ages, including the economically productive groups rather than the elderly. Survivors to old age, however, do very often suffer from eye diseases and blindness.

Trachoma

Trachoma is an almost universal infection—most prevalent in the poorer areas of the world, in the main in the developing countries, but quite widespread, for example, in backward communities within such an advanced country as Japan. In most areas where it prevails it co-exists over much of its range with the other two variables in Ida Mann's epigram cited earlier—blindness and malnutrition—and closely interacts with them. However, as she points out, trachoma does often seem to avoid the very poorly nourished, though they may have eye damage from such another cause as keratomalacia, spots spreading over the cornea, associated with vitamin A deficiency (and incidentally commoner after attacks by some such infection as typhoid).[7]

Trachoma is one of those diseases where the pathogenic organism has been known for many years but where there nevertheless is a case for essentially geographical analysis of its areal distribution pattern, and of the web of cultural and social and economic causes (even political ones)—in a single phrase, an ecologically based geography of trachoma. The studies known to me have been carried out not by a professional geographer but by an ophthalmologist of wide experience and repute, who has long been an enthusiastic practitioner of ophthalmological geography.[8] She is convinced of the importance of the human ecology and human geography of the disease, and proceeds essentially by comparing records of trachoma (and other eye diseases) from different countries and from different groups within particular countries (for instance, white and Aboriginal

Australians). The results are compelling, though her studies are quite different in approach from those of river blindness, in which professional geographers *have* been involved.

The trachoma organism, *Chlamydia trachomatis*, was isolated and cultivated in the laboratory by a group of workers in Pekin under T'ang,[9] and the experiment was confirmed in Australia by Ida Mann and Dorothy Perret in 1959. For some years after that the organism was fairly confidently regarded as a virus. From much earlier laboratory identification in 1912 the organism had been known to exist, and was variously named and attributed; Ida Mann's book refers to it as a virus and it has also been classified with the Rickettsiae organisms intermediate in size between bacteria and viruses, which include, for instance, the pathogen of scrub typhus. Recently opinion has veered back to placing it outside the viruses, because of its response to antibiotics and its apparent ability to synthesize its own protein; it is now placed among the *Bedsonia*, probably very small bacteria, along with the pathogens of psittacosis (parrot's disease) and lymphogranuloma venereum.

It has been said the disease is as old as poverty and overcrowding—for instance, in ancient Egypt and India.[10] Ida Mann's almost innumerable eye inspections and specimens, laboratory investigations and library correlations have shown that 100 years ago trachoma was widespread among white Australians, as it was in Europe at that time. On the other hand, her surveys show absence of the disease as a public-health problem now among white Australians and among the few very isolated Aborigines, and she was able to check these findings from very isolated tribal groups in New Guinea and elsewhere in Polynesia.

The final picture is of a spectrum of conditions varying from freedom from the disease in prosperous developed societies, to its increase with poverty, dirt, lack of hygiene and especially washing facilities and clean dust-free housing—dust and sand are a serious problem wherever housing is poor in many parts of Australia—and where people huddle together under poor conditions, as in many Aboriginal groups in shanty towns fringing country towns, and in many New Guinea groups in shanty towns and slums in and around Port Moresby and other towns.

However, the disease decreases again as one goes to comparatively untouched Aboriginal or tribal areas, and vanishes completely among extremely isolated groups.

The infection causes blindness in a proportion of cases, by causing lesions of the conjunctiva and cornea. Ida Mann's findings and synthesis of other work show that the trachoma infection proper is often, even normally, a comparatively mild and self-limiting disease. However, under conditions of poverty, dirt, prevalence of house flies and bush flies, and overcrowding, the infected eye is often further insulted by attacks by secondary infections from other bacteria, such as *Staphylococcus aureus* (the normally commensal 'nose germ', which occasionally causes boils and styes), or the Koch-Weeks bacillus (which causes 'pink eye'). In her own words: 'Western Australia's reputation as the land of sin, sand, sorrow and sore eyes rests on the prevalence among early settlers of trachoma and epidemic purulent ophthalmia. These two and possibly other infectious ophthalmias were, in the absence of accurate diagnosis, popularly known as 'sandy blight' and were a common experience in practically all country districts, especially in arid, fly-ridden areas.'

This historical picture led Ida Mann into a long and arduous series of journeys and eye surveys. A century before, trachoma was widespread in Australia, as indeed it was in contemporary Europe, but it has gradually diminished and died out as a serious public-health problem in prosperous and hygienic communities, where secondary eye infections are not common, even if the trachoma organism remains endemic. However, ophthalmic surveys in the Kimberley area of the north-west of Western Australia in the early 1950s revealed 1,200 cases in 3 months, 97 per cent in Aboriginal and 3 per cent in white people. Further surveys in the north-west yielded similar results, as did work in the eastern goldfields of Western Australia; in the Warburton Ranges, further from civilization, the disease was milder though still affecting over half the Aboriginal population. Further questions arose. Ida Mann asked:

Was it introduced by early settlers and gold prospectors? Or by Chinese, Malays or Afghans? Was it endemic in the country before its settlement? Owing to the universal distribution of the disease it was impossible to answer these questions from investigations in Australia alone. The nomadic habits of the aborigines in themselves could account for its spread. Older doctors mostly remembered times when it was much more prevalent among persons of European stock than it is now, and it seems possible, though quite unprovable, that it had been introduced to the natives by the first white settlers.

The study of an Aboriginal group that was not subject to European influence until trachoma had ceased to be important among white people might resolve the question. The opportunity arose not in the event with Australian Aboriginals but in New Guinea. Some areas there, like the Gazelle peninsula, had been opened up as early as 1875, but in contrast there were still isolated valleys with little or no contact with Europeans until very recently, and some had few exchanges even with the European-influenced coastal areas. The survey very strongly suggested that trachoma was not endemic, but introduced during earlier phases of European contact, and later contacts did not effect fresh introductions of the disease. By analogy Professor Mann is confident that trachoma in Australia is introduced, not endemic.

As early as 1688 Dampier and his pirate crew landed for 2 months in the King Sound area; this may link up with the substantial trachoma rates round Kimberley that first stimulated Dr Mann's investigations, though the picture is complicated by the importation last century of Chinese and Bengali labourers, almost certainly including trachoma sufferers. The Aboriginal population became severely infected, and have remained so because their standards of living and hygiene have not improved in pace with improvements among white people, a proportion of whom, however, also became infected, by trachoma and by secondary infections that do much of the damage to the eyes. The different degrees of contact with trachoma, and different ways of life and of standards of personal and community hygiene, yielded material for valuable analyses by Dr Mann:

We have been able to confirm that pure virus trachoma is a mild self-limiting disease which becomes serious, endangering sight, only when secondary infection occurs. This explains why it dies out when living conditions improve, why it is worse in the fly-ridden countries, why it is very mild when first introduced into healthy isolated highland or desert communities, and why its apparent clinical manifestations vary from an absolutely symptomless infection healing in the course of a year or two with negligible scars to a severe lifelong disability ending in blindness. By surveying this large and varied tract of country we have been able to observe all the intermediate stages (sometimes even in the same areas, for example, the Kimberleys) and to be certain that we are dealing with the same disease throughout. This has removed a lot of misconceptions on the diagnostic criteria of trachoma and partly explains the lack of notification in the past, since the tarsal plates would not be examined if the patient was not complaining, so all cases of 'trachoma pur' would be missed.

Ida Mann's findings are applicable throughout the enormous range of this overwhelmingly important disease. Readers who can find her popular travel book, *The Cockney and the Crocodile*, written under the name of Caroline Gye, are recommended to read it, and doubtless to fall under its spell.[11] It is not just another travel book; it is what one might call an eye-detective story!

Onchocerciasis or river blindness

Onchocerciasis is an important cause of eye disease, and of blindness in a proportion of those infected, in West and Central Africa and in Latin America from Mexico to Venezuela and Colombia. Onchocerciasis is named from a worm parasite on man (and only man on present knowledge), called *Onchocerca volvulus*. The adult female may be as long as 33–50cm, though only 270–400 microns in diameter (roughly 0·1–0·2mm), while the smaller male is about 2–4cm long by 130–210 microns in diameter.

Figure 36 shows the onchocerciasis cycle. The long-lived adult

82

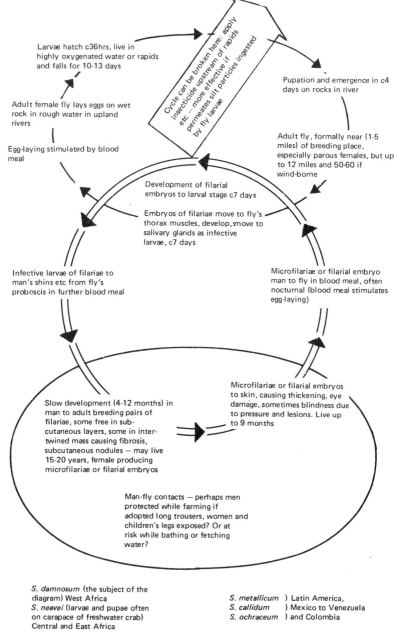

Figure 36. The river-blindness or onchocerciasis cycle.
(Source: Learmonth, A. T. A.)

worms live in an interlocked mass, round which the body develops a fibrous tissue or a fibrosis that forms distinctive nodules from pea size to golf ball size, beneath the skin. There may also be free adult filariae in the skin tissues. The diagram distinguishes these adult filariae from the microfilariae hatched out by egg-bearing adult females, which spread freely through the skin tissue, remaining there unchanged for up to 9 months, awaiting, as it were, the chance of being picked up by a bloodsucking black fly of a particular tropical species of the almost world-wide genus *Simulium*. (The vector species are noted in Figure 36.)

The microfilariae cause thickening of the skin; if this affects the eye, damage occurs, and possibly blindness develops through perforating blood vessels, pressure and inflammation.[12] On the other hand, some people seem able to generate immunity to the harmful effects; and a diet rich in vitamin A, found in palm oil, offers protection from blinding lesions, so that river blindness in West Africa belongs primarily to savannah rather than to the wetter oil palm tracts towards the coast.[13]

Focusing on river blindness on West Africa, and therefore on the vector species there, *Simulium damnosum*, we need only stress that breeding is concentrated on stretches of rapids and falls on upland rivers (over about 2,000ft or 600m). The fly preys largely on animals of various kinds, but feeds voraciously on people if man–fly contacts are close.

Treatment of the infection by drugs is possible, but needs skilled medical supervision and is apt to be unpleasant, so that mass therapy is not likely in developing countries at present. Prospects for eradication of the disease and of preventing much future blindness, therefore, are concentrated on this marked localization of the breeding places. It has been realized for some years that this localization makes it possible to treat breeding sites by insecticides. The volume of the river at a breeding site can be calculated, and a proportionate volume of an insecticide emulsion can be put in the river above the 'white water' of the rapids or falls used for breeding, allowing for the spreading out of the emulsion and its dispersion by turbulence. It is effective for up to 40 miles (64km) downstream, and moreover the insecticide is absorbed into silt particles upon which the black-fly larvae feed.

This knowledge has in the last few years been applied in a vast, complex, costly and imaginative project by the World Health Organization. It is hoped to speed both survey of 'white water' and of river volumes in the affected areas, allowing for changes in seasonal incidence, and also the application of insecticides by means of helicopters and light aircraft. Hovercraft were considered, but they were not sufficiently flexible to deal with all the different sizes of rivers and types of rapids and waterfalls encountered over such a vast part of the tropical world. The project is in progress and, though difficulties of both a technical and a financial nature are being met, this scourge may be one that can be dealt with by specific campaigns.

On the other hand, it would be possible to combat this disease, as so many others of the so-called 'tropical diseases', by the process of all-round social and economic development, including education. Since the black fly bites mainly the lower limbs, changes in dress or adaptations of work habits or bathing or water-carrying habits might well suffice, given understanding of the disease cycle. This depends on education, but not necessarily at an unattainable level; already there is evidence from Northern Ghana that for the first time the people are linking the disease specifically with the fly.[14] The social and ecological geography of river blindness have been studied by Hunter and by Bradley.[15]

Figure 37 shows the foci of black-fly breeding in northern Ghana. Breeding extends north into Upper Volta, but not much is found beyond 12°N. The black fly vanishes for some 6 months during the dry season, yet within hours of the first showers of the wet, it reappears in adult form. Hunter produced a primarily geographical hypothesis that these adult flies were in fact immigrant, moving north with the tropical maritime air—warm, humid and congenial to insect life—which brings the rains. This idea had not previously been investigated because the early rains come in depressions moving east to west, and the east seemed an unlikely source of immigrant flies, since conditions there are broadly similar. Hunter, however, suggested that since these east to west moving disturbances are in the nature of waves moving along the advancing front of tropical maritime air, adult flies could in fact be moving from more humid zones farther south

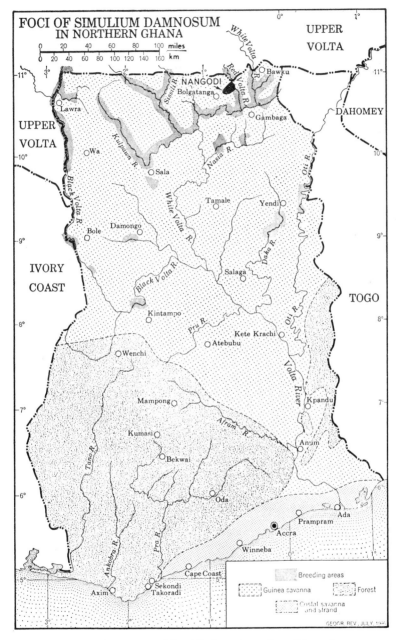

Figure 37. Foci of the vector of river blindness in northern Ghana, ie
Simulium or black fly. (Source: Hunter, J. M. 'River blindness in Nangodi,
Northern Ghana: a hypothesis of cyclical advance and retreat', *Geog Rev*, 56,
Fig 2, p 403.)

though caught up in easterly disturbances. Figure 36 noted the normal flight distance of *Simulium damnosum* as about 12 miles (20km) but extending up to some 60 miles (100km) when additional impetus is given by the wind. Subsequent research tends to support Hunter's hypothesis. His main contribution, however, was made as a human geographer, especially as settlement geographer studying human population and dwelling places over time. He wrote:

> When a house is abandoned, its roof timbers are usually removed ... so that within a few years the torrential wet-season rains wash its mud walls to the ground. As a result, evidence on the ground is easily overlooked. Air photographs, however, show no lack of evidence of former occupation. In more recently abandoned areas, nearer the present edge of settlement, traces of the typical radial system of footpaths can be seen. There is also evidence of sheetwash erosion in overcultivated areas now abandoned. In these areas tree growth is still restricted, decades later. But the clearest evidence lies in the different rates at which woody vegetation recolonizes abandoned farmland.... The area immediately around each house customarily received the greatest amount of manure; consequently when abandoned, it supports a more vigorous growth of natural vegetation. Clumps of thicker vegetation thus reveal former house sites, particularly where they contain baobab trees, which commonly serve as domestic shrines ...

Figure 38 shows very clearly the retreat of the frontier near Sakoti, a settlement about 3 miles west of a focus of black-fly breeding on the Red Volta river and chosen because of the availability of 1:10,000 air photographs, taken in 1949. After patient sifting of data and elimination of other main causes of the retreat, such as soil erosion or trypanosomiasis (sleeping sickness), Hunter was modestly confident of his conclusions.

Settlement once extended to the bank of the Red Volta, but has now retreated west by stages, still continuing, for abandonment of thirty-six houses was recorded from December 1949

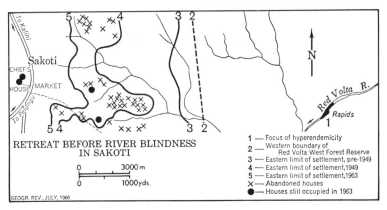

Figure 38. Retreat before river blindness in Sakoti, northern Ghana. Sakoti, immediately to the south of the Nangodi traditional area, was chosen by Hunter because of the availability of air photography of suitable date and scale to show the process of retreat from the river (it is known locally that settlement once extended to the bank of the river). In the area between lines 3 and 4 abandoned footpaths are visible on air photographs taken in December 1949 (scale 1:10,000), though most of the houses had washed away. Crosses between lines 4 and 5 (limit of settlement at time of Hunter's ground survey in April 1963) represent thirty-six houses abandoned during the $13\frac{1}{2}$-year period. Of the two houses shown as 'still occupied', the lower one is a resistant outlier of settlement, and the upper one was in process of being abandoned at the time of the survey. (Source: as Figure 37, Hunter, Fig 8.)

to April 1963. Discussion with village elders suggested that settlement was advancing on the bank of the Red Volta as late as about 1918. Hunter says:

We may calculate then, that around Gongo, north of the main road, settlement has retreated at a mean rate of one mile every seven years; south of the road around Nkunzesi and Nyaboka, where farmland has been relinquished more slowly, the mean rate is one mile every twelve to fourteen years. As farming declines, scrub and trees advance to recolonize the abandoned area, and game increases. The Nangodi-Naba's house in Kalini, once centrally situated, now stands at the eastern extremity of the chiefdom; this is true also of the Sakoti-Naba's house.

All along the retreating frontier of settlement there is a pervading atmosphere of decline and decay. Few of the houses are well maintained; although land is abundant, farms are not large and tend to be neglected because of limitations in the labour force, many of whom are blind. To the lay observer, nutritional standards seem to be low, and the incidence of minor infections, such as sores, is much higher than in the interior. When one visits these small, isolated, and dying communities, one cannot help feeling the contrast between the vigour and energy of the central and western sections, such as Soliga and Zanlerigu, and the lethargy and quiet resignation on the border of the blind area.

Hunter then went on to formulate an imaginative hypothesis that movements of the frontier of settlement like this, repeated over time and throughout the river-blindness tracts, might add up to a cyclic advance and retreat of the frontier. In earlier periods, of course, he had to take into account additional factors like slave raiding. He was able to sift oral tradition and compare, for instance, Forestry Department records with recent air photographs, and postulate a cycle of settlement from the late nineteenth century, when there was in-migration, motivated by dearth, from a wide area into empty riverside bush, some on the very banks of the river:

They prospered for a while, possibly for twenty to twenty-five years (1890–1895 to 1915–1918 approximately), and then disease began to take its toll, wiping out whole communities, weakening others, and reducing their capacity to work and to feed themselves adequately, so that slowly, inexorably, the process of abandonment came into operation. Beginning along the Red Volta, where the incidence of disease was greatest, land has been abandoned at the rate of one mile every seven to fourteen years for the past forty-five to fifty years. Nearly two-fifths of Nangodi has now been deserted, and the retreat continues. Although a combination of riverine diseases (including sleeping sickness) may be responsible for this retreat, the primary agent is, indisputably, river blindness.

In this instance the main thrust of geographical research —apart, that is, from the contribution towards solving the mystery of the sudden appearance of adult black fly with the first rains—assisted understanding of the broader significance of the disease for the whole community life, rather than discovering the disease cycle as such. This makes an important point: the human ecology and human geography of a disease may present baffling problems for years or decades after the mechanics of the pathogens and the vectors have been made clear.

Since Hunter wrote, further geographical work by Bradley has been going on in the Hawal valley in east central Nigeria, in a carefully designed research project, including control villages on uplands free of onchocerciasis except for returned temporary migrants to lowland and fly-infested areas. Initial studies of the entomological aspects suggested greater freedom of men than women and children from biting by *Simulium* because of their recent adoption of long trousers as common dress. However, risks at bathing and water-collecting by women and children might be lessened by some suggestion of dislike of wet skin by the biting fly. (Or is a slap from a wet hand more apt to kill a fly?) Studies of very simple indices of prosperity like house materials, utensils and furniture, show something of the economic impact of onchocerciasis. People with impaired sight travel shorter distances to farm, and therefore are progressively restricted, though even totally blind people do try to cultivate. Though communal help to the handicapped does operate, the total burden of gradually increasing dependency upon the population as a whole must be considerable.

The lowland villages subject to river blindness confirmed many of Hunter's hypotheses, despite the somewhat different grouping of the factors. Analysis of the age structure and residential or migration history proved particularly interesting. The average percentage of adults still living in the village of their birth differed markedly (7 per cent in lowland villages, 26 per cent in upland ones), as did their average ages (29 in lowland and 40 in upland villages). A clear picture emerges of the extension of settlement from relatively populous uplands into the population low-pressure area in the fly-infested lowlands, often followed by a retreat back to the uplands after 10 or 15 years. There is also movement of wives moving from the uplands into the lowlands on marriage, though there is increasing reluctance to marry men from lowland villages. (This may echo the movement, commented on by Daniel Defoe, of brides from the upland rim of the English fen country to ague-stricken (that is, malarious) fen villages.)

Desertion of villages does occur, and while fear of spirits is associated with several diseases other than river blindness, including smallpox and the dusty dry-season scourge of cerebrospinal meningitis, river blindness is associated with deserted villages both by deliberate evacuation from fear of 'spirits', more recently by fear of disease, and also by sheer attrition through death (as Hunter found in Ghana). That some people with years of man–fly contact did not succumb to the disease is suggestive of the immunity factor already noted, and this may repay further investigation. Are the differences due to differences in genetic factors, or diet? Are some families getting more vitamin A, for instance, or does metabolism differ significantly in this context?[16] The potential value of essentially geographical field survey in such work has perhaps been demonstrated.

A necessarily brief list of infectious diseases has been reviewed from a geographer's viewpoint: yellow fever, malaria, trachoma, onchocerciasis, infectious hepatitis and influenza, and except for trachoma it is reasonable to claim that geographers have made some contribution to understanding of the disease complex and sometimes suggested an approach to forecasting which might prove of practical use. Many other intriguing problems remain for geographical analysis. There is for instance what appears to be quite different behaviour by the same organisms or organisms at present indistinguishable from each other in the treponemal infections causing yaws (a non-venereal skin disease) especially in humid tropical areas, endemic syphilis (again non-venereal) especially in drier tropical areas, and venereal syphilis as an important social disease in developed and developing countries over a wide spectrum of climates. A distinguished natural historian of disease has suggested that treponemal skin infections may have become specialized as venereal infections, and his work is only one example of a number of works challenging conventional thinking about infectious diseases and the possibility of their abolition.[17]

This sort of world view of infections of man, or perhaps the constantly mounting number of viruses parasitic on man—probably many newly evolved or mutated rather than merely newly discovered—leads to the conclusion that in the end the eradication of infectious disease is unattainable. There may be exceptions—the eradication of smallpox has recently been claimed, and if the claim is justified by events we may well celebrate a major triumph for preventive medicine. But on the whole the problem is how best to live with infections, to reduce them to tolerable proportions as public-health problems, rather than to expend enormous resources on eradication projects that may well be predestined to failure.

CHAPTER FIVE

Some Apparently Non-infectious Diseases

Introduction

The title of this chapter, which deals with cancers and bronchitis, is not very clear-cut. It hedges, both because some cancers, for instance, now appear to be more related to infections and parasites than seemed likely a few years ago, and because there is blurring of classification in respect of bronchitis and several other apparently non-infectious diseases. Nevertheless there is a category of diseases that cannot at present be treated in the same spectrum as those discussed in Chapters 2–4. The developed world looms larger in this chapter, because of the greater importance of such diseases there now that most infections have been reduced in importance, at least as causes of death and serious illness. Conversely, most people in the Third World do not live long enough to die of diseases like cancer, several important forms of which are causes of mortality in the middle-aged and the old rather than among young people.

In relation to such diseases it is more difficult to see patterns in common, except for the truism that we must all die of something, and increasingly in developed countries it is likely to be from heart or vascular collapse, or cancer of some form. At present neither the ecological nor the spatial patterns of these diseases appear to hang together in the same way as those of the infectious diseases, though with increasing knowledge this may change. Nevertheless there are interesting ecological and spatial patterns, and in some ways the intellectual challenges may be the greater when insights are partial—when 'we see in part and we prophesy in part'.

Cancers

Cancer is a disorder wherein cell growth is no longer coordinated with the need for new cells, generating a colony of relatively undifferentiated cells that draw on the body's supply of nutrients but contribute nothing, and in time outnumber the healthy cells in their neighbourhood. Mutations that cause cells to divide in this way can result from a number of factors: ionizing radiation, which is also used in treatment; carcinogens, the most widespread being in tobacco smoke; possibly following virus infection, though none has yet been positively identified with human cancer. Moreover heredity may predispose people to cancer. There are marked regional differences in the occurrence of cancers, sometimes over very small distances; some of these have plausible explanations, while others, such as the fact that cancer of the rectum is twice as common in Denmark as Norway, have not, though there an association with heavy beer drinking is suspected.

Even in the brief definition above it has become clear that there is a geographical distribution of cancers that varies a good deal, apparently, for cancers of different sites—the geography of lung cancer differs from that of stomach cancer, from that of liver cancer, and so on. These differences can be pursued on the world scale: for instance, cancer of the lung is at present a disease mainly of temperate and developed countries, and cancer of the liver mainly of tropical and developing countries. A recent publication from the Vrije Universiteit of Brussels makes it possible to illustrate some of these differences. I have selected just three of the maps from this work, drawn on a demographic base.

Figure 39 shows the proportion of cancer to total mortality; there is a heavy preponderance in the developed world including North America, temperate Latin America, Australia and New Zealand, Japan and much of Europe but not the USSR. The pattern cannot be accounted for solely by longer life in the high cancer countries, though that is an important factor in contrasts between the developed world and the Third World. Figure 40 portrays the male mortality for cancers of the trachea, bronchus

94

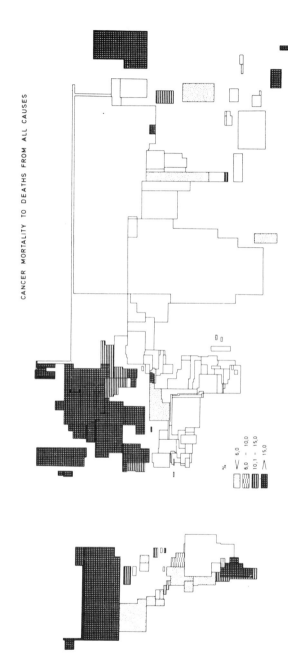

CANCER MORTALITY TO DEATHS FROM ALL CAUSES

Figure 39. World map, ratio of cancer mortality to total mortality. (Source: Geografisch Instituut, Vrije Universiteit, Brussels, 1975.)

95

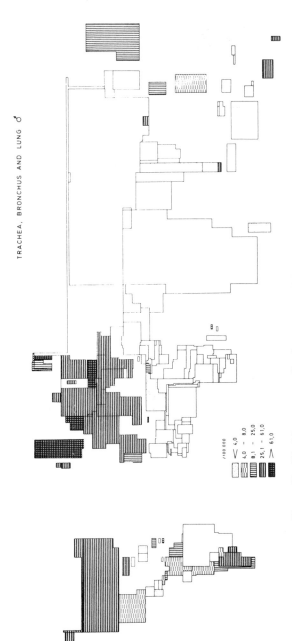

TRACHEA, BRONCHUS AND LUNG ♂

/100 000

< 4,0
4,0 - 8,0
8,1 - 25,0
25,1 - 61,0
> 61,0

Figure 40. World map, mortality from cancer of the trachea, lung and bronchus, males. (Source: as Figure 39.)

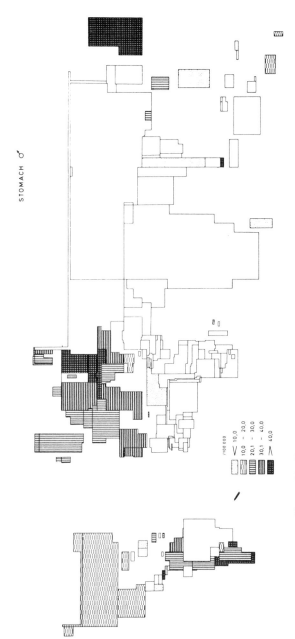

Figure 41. World map, mortality from cancer of the stomach, males. (Source: as Figure 39.)

and lung, and Figure 41 that for male cancers of the stomach. While these two maps echo the pattern of Figure 39, since they are responsible for a considerable proportion of the mortality it shows, they are also contrasted. Note, for instance, the greater weight of north-western Europe for lung cancers, of eastern Europe for cancer of the stomach. Australia and New Zealand resemble north-western Europe in this, while Japan is more like eastern Europe. Singapore and Hong Kong seem to be entering the developed world in this unenviable respect, while Sri Lanka shows significant stomach cancer, a feature more detailed mapping would show it shares with south-western India, where local diets, perhaps condiments or ways of chewing the areca nut and betel vine leaf mixture with tobacco, have long been under suspicion as carcinogenic. Evidence about the role of radioactive minerals in coastal sands in Kerala in India is conflicting.

The corresponding maps for cancer of the breast and of the cervix uteri (not illustrated in this book) show somewhat analogous contrasts—breast cancer is more important in north-western Europe, cervical cancers in eastern Europe, while Japan has moderate incidence of both. Yet Japanese populations in the United States, for instance, seem gradually to approximate to US patterns, suggesting that there are environmental factors at work: in fact at present a proportion of 80 per cent of cancers as due to environmental factors, to 20 per cent genetic, is often quoted.

Later in the chapter you will find some studies at a medium scale of particular cancers within Britain, for instance, or of some in particular countries or tracts of Africa. One or two are essentially geographical in approach, like that by Allen-Price in Devon (Figure 42). He showed that in the village of Horrabridge, for instance, the area north of the River Walkham had one-third of deaths due to cancer, compared with 1 in 12 in adjacent parts of the village regarded as homogeneous in all known aspects of community life, except that the source of water supply was different; and he was convinced enough to campaign successfully for an appropriate change in the water supply.[1]

It was well known to nineteenth-century workers that cancers in Britain (and elsewhere) showed marked regional differences, and the distribution patterns were mapped;[2] however, data did

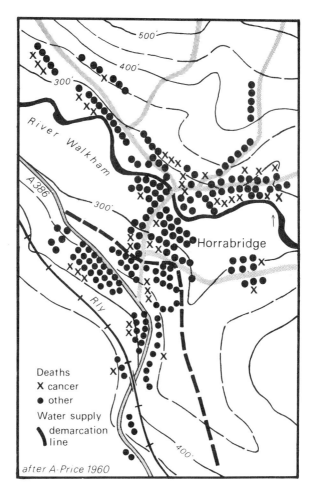

Figure 42. Cancer mortality in Horrabridge, Devon. Cancer deaths and
deaths from other causes mapped in relation to three sources of water supply
(i) north of the River Walkham, (ii) between the Walkham and the pecked line,
and (iii) south and west of the pecked line. (Source: Allen-Price, E. D. 'Uneven
distribution of cancer in West Devon with particular reference to the divers
water supplies', *Lancet*, 1, 1960.)

not permit detailed differentiation of the type of cancer, so that the
maps remained at an illustrative level, informing the interested
general practitioner, for instance, of the life or death chances his
patients might have in the Lake District as compared with East
Anglia. Interest was renewed with some serious geographical
analysis in the early 1950s, not, however, immediately followed
up.[3] The crucial paper on cigarette smoking and lung cancer drew

a great deal of attention in the late 1950s;[4] indeed a slight fall in total lung-cancer deaths may arise partly from this concern, reducing mortality in the middle-aged 20 years later—mortality in women, however, is still rising. But this after all was only one cancer, and even here there were puzzling features—the mapped mortality rates did not seem to correspond with a map of cigarette smoking, as Sir Dudley Stamp pointed out at the London meeting of the International Geographical Union in 1964 (see Figure 43).

About the same time as Sir Richard Doll was working on tobacco smoking and cancer Percy Stocks was working on cancer and bronchitis mortality in relation to atmospheric deposits,[5] and in emphasizing high urban incidence he suggested that pollution of food by urban smoke might account for high urban rates—not only for lung cancer but for stomach cancer also.

From the geographer's viewpoint and about the same period Professor G. M. Howe, one of whose maps has already been used as Figure 44, was becoming interested in the geography of disease, initially from a chance encounter with the distinctive geography of cancer of the stomach in Wales, and then extending his interest to the whole of the UK and to the whole of the available mortality data to produce the two editions of the *National Atlas of Disease Mortality.*[6]

Howe's maps are based on standardized mortality ratios, so that they show 'over-representation' or 'under-representation' of, say, lung-cancer mortality in a particular area as compared with the national expectation of mortality from that cause after allowing for the age and sex structure of the local population. (This is done by dividing the actual deaths in the area by the number that would have occurred if the death rates for each age and sex group had been the same as the rates for the country as a whole; and then expressing the result as a percentage, so that an area with exactly the same as the national expectation of mortality has a ratio of 100, while areas 'over-represented' in, say, lung cancers have higher ratios, and areas 'under-represented' have ratios below 100.) Moreover the 1970 atlas presented data according to a 'demographic base' map, which prevents over-emphasis on areas like North Wales, where populations are small; and the

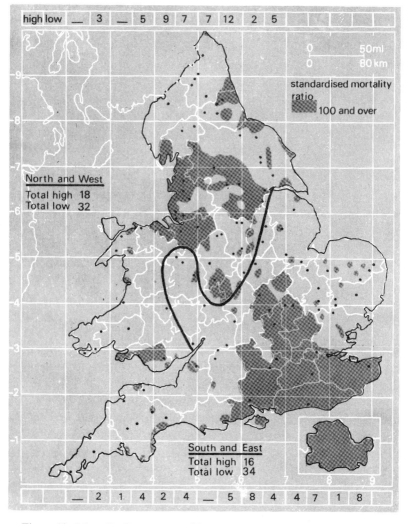

Figure 43. Mortality from cancer of the trachea, lung and bronchus, males, 1954–58. This is clearly not one of the distribution patterns suggesting disadvantageous conditions in the North and West of England and Wales I have hypothesized in discussing several other maps in this series, eg Figures 50 and 51 of bronchitis mortality. This is confirmed by the χ^2 test. (Source: Howe G. M. *National Atlas of Disease Mortality*, RGS/Nelson, 1970; Open University, *D203 Decision making in Britain*, Block 5, *Health*, Bletchley, Open University Press, 1972, Fig 12, pp 46–7.)

1970 maps also distinguish the areas where the regional differences can be regarded as 'statistically significant'—that is, unlikely to have arisen by chance fluctuations.

These maps, based on places of residence at death and grouped by administrative units, are as refined as we can expect, at least until new methods of presenting data not related to administrative areas become available—for instance, mapping by rectangular grid squares of 1 × 1km in rural areas and 100 × 100m in urban areas, as provided for in the 1971 census. Howe's maps should be taken seriously, though one cannot say that they have been very intensively followed up, or that they have produced any major discoveries about the causes of particular cancers. The maps reproduced here often cover England and Wales only, but we shall refer to the mapping done for Scotland, Northern Ireland and the Isle of Man whenever that throws further light on a particular disease pattern.

Let us start where Professor Howe began, with cancer of the stomach. In Figure 44 (females for the period 1954–58) one is struck by the concentration of high rates in a great swathe running across both rural and urban Wales and the north and north-west of England, with an extension into the West Midlands industrial conurbation. There is a group of high rates around the fen country in Kesteven, Northamptonshire and Bedford. Elsewhere high rates are mainly urban, including some very high ones in some London boroughs. The picture from Scotland and Northern Ireland is broadly consistent with this pattern, as is the map for the period 1959–63, with some exceptions—the counties round the Fens, for instance, do not show such consistently high rates. For both periods the maps for males show broadly similar trends.

The disadvantage of the north and west of the British Isles in relation to stomach cancers is clear; many of the differences are statistically significant. The suggestion by Stocks that pollution of food by urban smoke might be causal receives some support from the widespread patterns of high urban rates, even in quite small towns; but it cannot be regarded as proved, since urban and rural populations alike appear on the maps over much of the north and west of England and Wales. Professor P. J. Lawther has

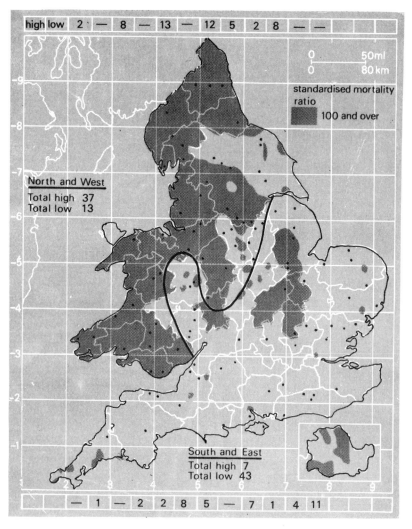

Figure 44. Cancer of the stomach, females, 1954–58. Many readers may be surprised at the strong suggestion of higher risks in the North and West of England and Wales, and in the East Midlands. This is confirmed by the χ^2 test, with a probability of 99·9 per cent. (Source: as Figure 43, Howe, 1970, p 37.)

suggested that smoke inside houses, especially in houses with old-fashioned open cooking and heating grates, might be a cause. So might smoked food, which has been under suspicion in areas of high stomach cancer in Iceland; bacon contains small quantities of carcinogenetic nitrosamines. There can scarcely be a genetic cause, over so wide and heterogeneous an area.

Diet may well be different in these north-west and western tracts than in the generally more prosperous south and east, but then there are the high urban rates of much of the south and east. Is there a dietetic factor? Scotland's diet in recent years has been high in margarine, cakes and biscuits, and beef; that of Wales in butter; that of the north of England (east and west) in margarine; and the Midlands' in pork.[7] Indications, therefore, are of a multivariate rather than a single-variable problem, though the problem is one very well worth probing further, taking due regard to factors that may have changed in a way significant for the future of disease—for instance, domestic smoke may have become less important in urban pollution, but car exhausts more so.

Lung cancer (Figure 43) is differently distributed. In England and Wales there is a cluster of high rates in the north-east, then a great belt in urban North Wales and in industrial Lancashire and Yorkshire; this is continued intermittently through the Midlands, especially the West Midlands conurbation, to link with a major concentration in Greater London and the south-east, with very high rates in many London boroughs. Elsewhere in England and Wales the high rates are mainly urban, except in South Wales, where, however, rates are lower for females than in the 1959–63 maps. The maps for females generally reflect the same broad patterns. Industrial and urban Scotland and Northern Ireland are consistent with this picture, as are, in very broad terms, the 1959–63 maps.

Is differential cigarette smoking to be supposed, say between town and country? Differences have been pointed out between Scotland and England and Wales, Scotsmen smoking 11 per cent more than their southern neighbours, and Scotswomen 15 per cent more, and smoking fewer tipped cigarettes.[8] But are like differences to be expected between, say, Cumberland–Northumberland and Lancashire–Yorkshire? If not, then we must expect that some factor other than cigarette smoking is seriously at work exacerbating the carcinogenetic effect of tobacco—probably urban pollution. As we noted earlier, urban pollution is changing, and while the effects of past smoke pollution will be in evidence for some time, the impact of increased exhaust-fume pollution will have to be considered. Again the patterns on the map, many significant on statistical testing, do seem worthy of wider recognition and also as justifying further research to complement all the effort put into identifying the relation between cancer and cigarette smoking.

The two cancers of women, cancer of the uterus and cancer of the breast, offer contrasted patterns (Figures 45 and 46). Cancer of the uterus is mainly a disease of the north and west of England and Wales (with some areas much less affected), and of areas in the south and east that one might regard as backward rural areas in terms of washing facilities etc, at least until recently. Such facilities have been mapped and there is evidence for this view. The same tendency can be seen from Scotland, Northern Ireland and the Isle of Man, and from the 1959–63 map. The tentative views of some epidemiologists that this cancer is related to poor penile and vaginal hygiene seems to be borne out, and these maps ought to be widely known and health education suitably pointed.

The patterns of breast cancer, while again slightly suggestive of rural areas being backward in baths etc, shows much more evenly balanced risks between much of Wales, the industrial north and west, and the Midlands, on the one hand, and the south and east of England on the other. Most of Northern Ireland seems to be lightly affected, but much of Scotland, urban and rural, has high rates. The 1959–63 map, however, shows some change, rates being lower in the industrial north and north-west of England and much of Wales, and in the industrial west of Scotland (though there the differences do not reach statistically significant levels, and could result from random or chance fluctuations in deaths from this cause).

Over whole populations this cancer is thought to be commoner among women who have not suckled babies than among those who have, though data are conflicting. (Rates tend to be low in

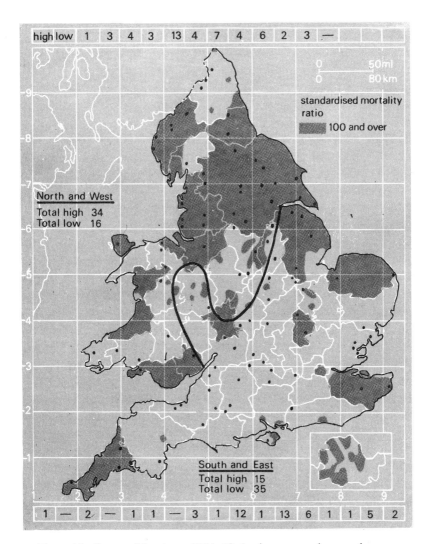

high low	1	3	4	3	13	4	7	4	6	2	3	—

standardised mortality ratio

100 and over

North and West

Total high 34
Total low 16

South and East
Total high 15
Total low 35

1	—	2	—	1	1	—	3	1	12	1	13	6	1	1	5	2

Figure 45. Cancer of the uterus, 1954–58. Again many readers may be surprised at the main spread of very high ratios in the North and West of England and Wales, though there are some also in parts of London and some medium-high rates in many more rural parts of the South and East, possibly linked with backward conditions of hygiene. The higher risks in the North and West are confirmed by the χ^2 test, at a probability of 99 per cent. (Source: as Figure 43, Howe, 1970, p 31.)

106

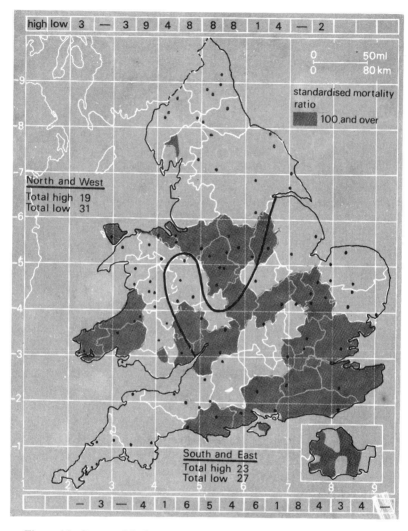

| high low | 3 | — | 3 | 9 | 4 | 8 | 8 | 8 | 1 | 4 | — | 2 |

0   50ml
0   80 km

standardised mortality
ratio
100 and over

North and West
Total high 19
Total low 31

South and East
Total high 23
Total low 27

| — | 3 | — | 4 | 1 | 6 | 5 | 4 | 6 | 1 | 8 | 4 | 3 | 4 | — |

Figure 46. Cancer of the breast, 1959–63. On visual inspection, this, like
Figure 46 of lung cancer, does not show the North and West as particularly at
risk, and this is confirmed by the χ^2 test. (Source: as Figure 43, Howe in Open
University, 1972, Fig 14, p 48.)

developing countries and in Latin America, and the more industrialized countries that have the higher rates. Of course variables other than breast feeding may be acting.) Further work on regional differences and any changes in incidence and in breast feeding may be justified, but at this stage no widespread educational or publicity campaign of the type indicated for cancer of the uterus need be contemplated. Such an epidemiological or geographical approach, of course, represents only one among many complementary efforts being made to understand a disease like breast cancer. Some recent work suggests that it may prove to be one of the cancers activated by a virus and, should this be confirmed, the geographical differences would have to be reassessed to see if they remain merely interesting or if they are still worth further analysis in greater depth than existing studies.

Professor Howe has followed up his two atlases of disease mortality for Britain, published in 1963 and 1970, with research on some items in greater analytical depth than the atlas format could justify. Continuing research can also be demonstrated in relation to cancers from my own much simpler and cruder atlases of disease mortality in Australia, also using standardized mortality ratios based on the excellent records available there.[9]

The lung-cancer mapping from those studies was followed up experimentally to a limited extent for a single state, Victoria (Figure 47). In that figure (a) is an isopleth or contour map, fairly straightforward if one is prepared to accept the conventions of mapping 'hills' and 'valleys' of cancer mortality, and those based on 'bench marks' consisting of standardized mortality ratio values placed in the geometric centre of each census and cancer recording district. On the other hand, Figure 47(b) is less a map and more a model, for further abstraction and generalization have been attempted; a very simple arithmetical method was used to produce 'generalized contours' by analogy with the geomorphologist's use of these—or with more mathematically sophisticated 'trend surface maps'. The initial aim was to produce a broad regional trend; this took a simple 'ridge' form, running and narrowing from south to north across the state. This was in itself suggestive of some relations with urban and industrial conditions, but there followed two further stages, in (c) and (d), showing

108

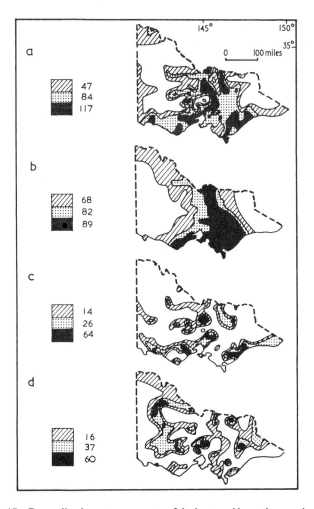

Figure 47. Generalized contours, cancer of the lung and bronchus, males, Victoria, Australia, 1961–64.

(a) Standardized mortality ratios mapped as isopleths, taking the geometrical centre of statistical divisions as 'spot-heights' and interpolating contours.
(b) Generalized contours based on 'spot-heights' at the same points, each averaging the set of values falling within a circle of 10,000sq miles (26,000km²) based upon each point; a map of regional trends.
(c) Positive anomalies based on a comparison of maps A and B.
(d) Negative anomalies based on a comparison of maps A and B. (Source: Learmonth, A. T. A. 'Atlases in medical geography', in McGlashan, N. D. [ed]. *Medical geography: techniques and field studies*, Methuen/University Paperbacks, 1972, Fig 10.6, p 143.)

respectively areas with positive and negative anomalies: mortality ratios were, in (c), above the broad regional contoured surface portrayed in (b), and below it in (d). This study was not followed up, so far as I am aware, for some years, partly because I left Australia, but recently I learned that the approach, duly refined from the crude experimental stage, may be tried in Tasmania, along with detailed use of the cancer registry and interviewing techniques, with the particular aim of throwing light on possible explanations for the positive and negative anomalies.[10]

Figure 39 illustrated dramatically the greater relative importance of cancer in the low mortality rates of the developed world, as compared with their small proportion of the high mortality rates of the Third World. However, it was noted that some cancers, such as cancer of the liver, are more important proportionately in developing countries than in developed ones. Other locally important cancers are cancer of the oesophagus and the cancer of the lymphatic system known as Burkitt's tumour, and geographical analysis of these has been used in Africa.

McGlashan used a combination of cartographic and statistical analysis of admittedly crude data to bring out a possible relation between cancer of the oesophagus and particular types of African alcoholic spirits (Figures 48 and 49). The type of still used varies regionally, and at first metal contamination was suspected, though not proved. Then a constituent of certain fermentation processes called nitrosamine came under suspicion; biochemical assays have not so far proved sufficiently consistent to justify a claim that the cause of the cancer has been identified by initially geographical investigation, but the work is continuing. The correlation seems clear enough, and for the moment it can only be suggested that repeated insult of throat tissues by crude alcohol are damaging. Indeed high local incidence of the same cancer in France may be related to the cider-based spirit calvados; a recent medical geography of the south of France includes important analyses of interrelations of cancers and alcoholism in France and in the generally temperate Midi.[11] However, the problem may go deeper than that. McGlashan has visited the southern shore of the Caspian, where there is high incidence of this cancer, particularly in women, which is unusual; he has suggested

110

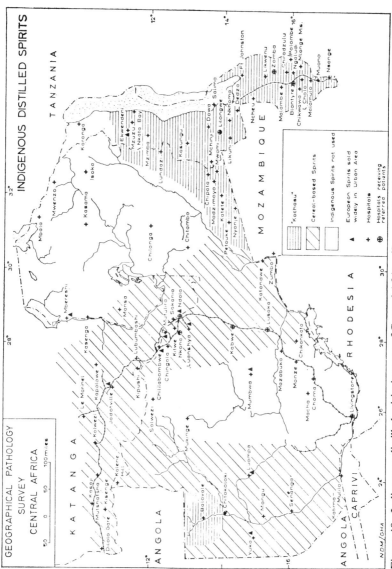

Figure 48. Indigenous distilled spirits in parts of Central Africa. (Source: McGlashan, N. D. 'Food Contaminants and Oesophageal Cancer' in McGlashan, 1972.)

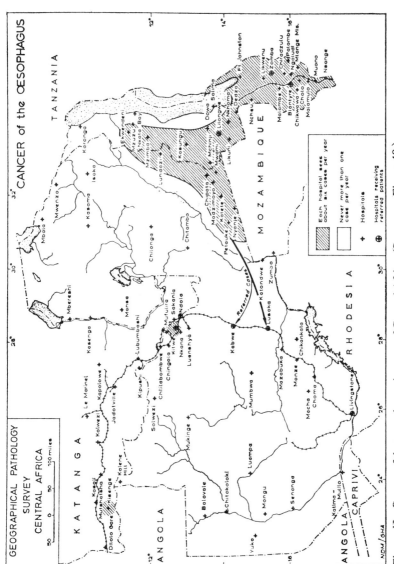

Figure 49. Cancer of the oesophagus in parts of Central Africa. (Source: as Figure 48.)

investigation of two items of food—one a local vinegar, the other a fermented preparation used as a tonic by pregnant and lactating women. In USSR rates are similarly high around the Caspian, but also in Yakutia and in Kazakhstan (where the consumption of boiling-hot tea is a suspected cause).

Burkitt's lymphoma was mapped in the early 1960s, by Burkitt himself, and he suggested that since the distribution pattern seemed to exclude high altitudes free from many biting arthropods, the cancer might be arthropod-borne or caused by an arthropod-borne virus or 'arbovirus'. This initial mapping and cartographic correlation was criticized as over-simplified, and later work by a geographer and a surgeon produced much more refined maps.[12] Various streams of research have converged on blood-group analysis, on apparent wavelike movement of fresh cases of the lymphoma, and possible relations with waves of malaria moving across forest and scrub country in a way not uncommon in parasitic diseases of forest terrain. It now seems possible that the lymphoma may be related to arthropod-borne disease, but to malaria rather than to an arbovirus.

Bronchitis

Bronchitis is simply inflammation of the air passages of the lungs. It may be either acute (normally a mild and fairly easily treated condition) or chronic (often defined arbitrarily as prevailing for over 3 months of the year). It is the chronic ailment that is regarded as 'the English disease', causing some 35,000 deaths a year in the United Kingdom, almost 1 per 1,000 of the total male population but only 0.4 per 1,000 of the females. These are higher rates than in other apparently comparable western countries, such as Norway or the USA, but, as we shall see, some of the disparity may be due to differences in diagnosis.

Before discussing chronic bronchitis further we should note two other conditions: (1) bronchiectasis, comparatively rare in western countries since the introduction of antibiotic drugs, and an irreversible sequel to a severe infection such as whooping cough in which the bronchi lose their elasticity and so their ability to clear themselves of mucus secretion; and emphysema, strictly pulmonary emphysema, in which prolonged severe coughing, often due to chronic bronchitis, has irreversibly increased the air spaces in the lungs at the expense of the lung tissue, so impairing its functions. Bronchiectasis is more often a separate entity from bronchitis, whereas emphysema, when it occurs, is commonly a sequel to it.[13]

The fundamental feature of bronchitis is that the inflammation of the bronchi causes excessive production of mucus secretion, and a normal function is deranged. The severity of the inflammation varies; it seems that it often starts with simple irritation or insult to the tissue, often from industrial smoke pollution, or quite possibly more often from the domestic smoke pollution of an open domestic heating or cooking fire. Even more commonly, it now seems, the cause is tobacco smoking, especially of cigarettes. This initial inflammation seems to permit normally harmless commensal organisms to become pathogenic infections.

These organisms include the following bacteria: *Haemophilus influenzae*, also a cause of pneumonia and occasionally meningitis when resistance is lowered by the influenza virus; the streptococcus *Pneumococcus*, another cause of pneumonia; the normally harmless and commensal organism of the intestines *Escherichia coli*; and *Staphylococcus pyogenes*, more familiar as a common cause of boils. If the effects of the initial insult and one or more infections become chronic, there may be a sequence of progressively more severe bronchitis: (1) simple chronic bronchitis, in which the patient coughs up clear mucus, since the specialized pear-shaped 'goblet' epithelial or skin cells of the mucous membrane are over-stimulated and over-produce; (2) chronic mucopurulent bronchitis, in which bacterial infection causes the discharge to be an opaque, often yellowish, mucopurulent sputum; and (3) chronic obstructive bronchitis, in which persistent coughing, irritation, and infection cause narrowing of the air passages and impairment of breathing.

At this stage, or even stage 2, the hairlike cilia are unable to move because of the over-production of mucus and pus, and become smoothed over; normal disposal of the mucus by swallowing with the saliva cannot operate; and only continued coughing—which accentuates the insult to the bronchi—can relieve the excess mucopurulent discharge.[14]

Antibiotics are useful against the bacterial organisms in reducing the severity rather than the number of attacks; influenza vaccination can reduce some of the risks; breathing exercises and efforts to stop smoking can help; and in severe air pollution various filters can be used. These are only palliatives and the high death rates in Britain and the high incidence of obstructive bronchitis, compared with, say, Norway and the USA, justify further discussion.

Some of the international disparities may be due to differences in diagnosis, for the field is a notoriously difficult one, and it is possible that many advanced cases may be diagnosed overseas as bronchiectasis and possibly emphysema. Even so, the differences do seem to be genuine. Smoking is presumably common, but smoking habits may differ—British cigarette smokers notoriously smoke their cigarettes to a very short butt compared with Americans—and also the rise of cigarette smoking may be differently phased; in Britain both cigarette consumption and bronchitis seem to have increased after 1920, in Norway after 1940. Large non-smoking groups like the Seventh Day Adventists in the USA have lower incidence of bronchitis (and of lung cancers also) than the general population.

Peter Wingate the author of the Penguin *Medical Encyclopaedia* points with some confidence to the combination of the British open coal fire and the chilly British bedroom as joint differentiating factors—initial irritation followed by the stimulus to coughing of the sharp change in temperature. The reader may recall from the discussion of lung cancer Professor P. J. Lawther's suspicions about the role of internal pollution from open fires and especially open cooking grates. As with cigarette smoking, the two very different respiratory disorders may share a good deal in their environmental relations. These differences in life style would account for smaller incidence in the south-east, where central heating must have spread much earlier than in the north, or Scotland, or Wales, or Northern Ireland, but if it plays a crucial role, changes should now be occurring as central heating becomes more widespread. Overcrowding has been suggested as more important than external air pollution, in Newcastle-upon-Tyne, for instance, and some geographical studies cited later will add to this. Inherited differences between, say, Welsh and English seem to be disproved, but may be significant in low incidence among negroes, even those who smoke; negro populations in Guyana, for example, are less susceptible than are the East Indians.

The disease tends to be commoner in men than in women, in the proportion of about 2 to 1 in Britain. This may relate to smoking—in men the risk is increased fivefold, in women only in those smoking more than a packet of cigarettes a day.

Lower socio-economic ratings seem to be associated with higher incidence, and downward social mobility has been invoked—that is, where bronchitis patients have moved into a lower social class than that of their father. Dusty jobs, including coalmining, have, not surprisingly, been incriminated. In Britain the disease seems to increase with age, say at and beyond middle-age, perhaps because of the cumulative effect of air pollution plus smoking, but this does not happen in the USA. The English disease accounts for a considerable absence from work: for example, almost 14 days per year in a local-authority staff of about 1,200 people, representing a loss of some 70 man-years. If multiplied up for the working community, the loss of production to the country as a whole must be considerable. However, there are regional differences in bronchitis, where the geographical contribution may emerge, so let us turn to these.

In Howe's map of bronchitis mortality for males in England and Wales in 1954–58 there is a concentration north of the Humber–Severn line of the higher rates—above national expectation of bronchitis mortality, itself high by international standards (Figure 50). The maps for male and for female mortality have a general family resemblance, but female mortality in 1954–58, though only some 43 per cent of male mortality, was so clearly concentrated in our north and west region, that Figure 51 is included for the benefit of readers not used to detailed analysis of maps. There are exceptions in the south and east of England, west of the Wash, in London (particularly in east and north-east boroughs), and in some smaller urban areas.

The 1959–63 data are statistically significant. The most northerly English counties are not among the most severely affected, though Tyneside is high; however, in Scotland rates are

116

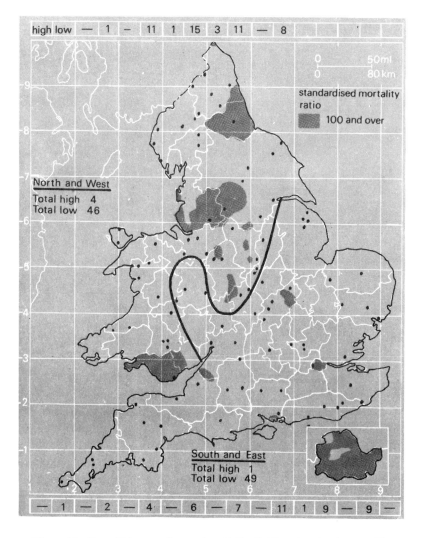

high low — 1 – 11 1 15 3 11 — 8

standardised mortality ratio
■ 100 and over

North and West
Total high 4
Total low 46

South and East
Total high 1
Total low 49

— 1 — 2 — 4 — 6 — 7 — 11 1 9 — 9 —

Figure 50. Bronchitis mortality, males, 1959–63. There is a dominance of low rates in our North and West regions, and the only appearance of high rates in our South and East regions is in parts of London. The South and East high total of 1 is too small a sample, so the χ^2 test cannot be used, but the map remains highly suggestive. (Source: Howe in Open University. *D203 Decision making in Britain*, Block 5, Bletchley, Open University Press, 1972, figure 9, p 42.)

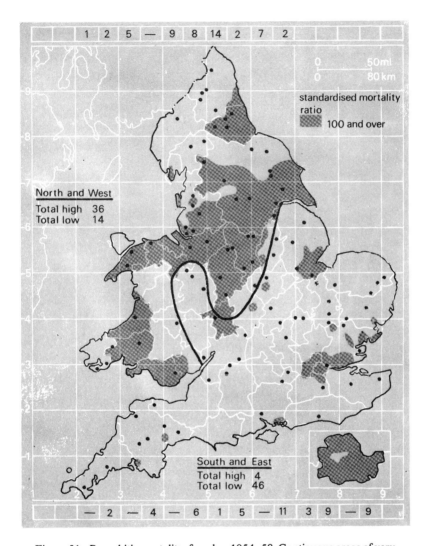

Figure 51. Bronchitis mortality, females, 1954–58. Contiguous areas of very high rates are strikingly concentrated in the North and West rather than in the South and East, with the very notable exception of parts of London. The χ^2 test cannot be applied to our sample totals of high and low for the two major regions, but the North and West bias is certainly strong. However, for 1959–63 (not illustrated here) a much larger proportion of high rates are found in London and the South East. (Source: as Figure 50.)

much lower in general, though to be sure there are some high rates in the mid Lowlands, particularly in Glasgow and other industrial areas. Northern Ireland and the Isle of Man seem to resemble Scotland rather than northern England. This may well be a matter of different practice in entering a cause of mortality on death certificates, rather as was suggested as a partial explanation of the contrast between death rates in the UK and those in Norway. It may be that more Scottish than English doctors quote the terminal or proximate cause of death, say pneumonia or more probably heart failure (though pneumonia also tends to fall off going north over the border).

The map of England and Wales would certainly suggest that cigarette smoking, unless it is heavier north of the Humber–Severn line, must be less important in regional contrasts than some factors connected with nineteenth-century industrial towns and cities, as distinct from the now more prosperous urban areas associated with light and service industries in the south and east of the country. Air pollution must certainly play its part, either in the external environment or related to the domestic coal fire and perhaps the chilly bedroom, as suggested by Peter Wingate. But if so, should not women on the whole be more affected than men, since they spend rather more time at home, and not less affected, as they generally are? Overcrowding may certainly play a major part, though high densities of population per dwelling or per room ought also to affect women if anything more than men. So far the problem may be thought to be due to a combination of causes—perhaps work in older industrial premises, combined with external and internal air pollution; overcrowding at home, work and leisure, in pubs and clubs; perhaps poor or periodically poor nutrition or heavy stress of anxiety over unemployment; and generally poor conditions of work and living, with little fresh air and enjoyable exercise.

Let us turn to two more detailed geographical studies. The first is multi-disciplinary, for it includes meteorological as well as geographer-climatologists' research, and it is also now quite an old study; but it is a classic one, and one that perhaps marked the end of an era in relation to smoke pollution in London.

Figure 52 shows one way of representing the great London

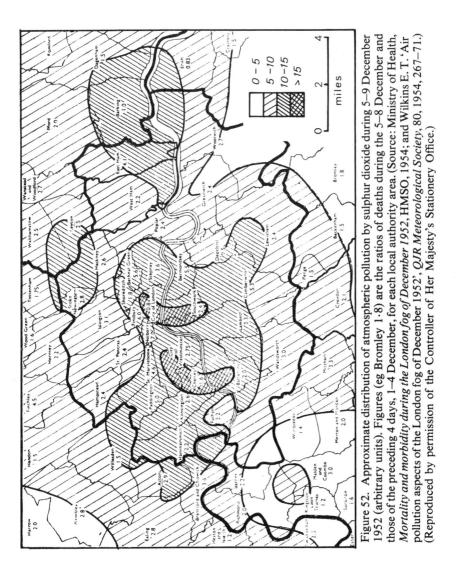

Figure 52. Approximate distribution of atmospheric pollution by sulphur dioxide during 5–9 December 1952 (arbitrary units). Figures (eg Bromley 1·8) are the ratios of deaths during the 5–8 December and those of the preceding 4 days, 1–4 December, for each local authority area. (Source: Ministry of Health, *Mortality and morbidity during the London fog of December 1952*, HMSO, 1954; and Wilkins E. T. 'Air pollution aspects of the London fog of December 1952', *QJR Meteorological Society*, 80, 1954, 267–71.) (Reproduced by permission of the Controller of Her Majesty's Stationery Office.)

smog of 5–9 December 1952 (by the sulphur dioxide pollution), to which were attributed at least 4,000 deaths and much illness. The daily concentration of smoke and of sulphur dioxide was very closely correlated with the increase in deaths, with the 'excess' deaths evidently due to the smog over the period, though death rates stayed abnormally high for some weeks afterwards as people succumbed to bronchitis, pneumonia or perhaps to complications developing during their illness or as their strength waned. Figure 52 also shows that the areal distribution of death rates shows higher rates generally in the highly polluted areas, though borough boundaries do not, of course, correspond with the 'contours' of pollution density. This great killing smog is not without its parallels. Many London smogs may well have gone unrecorded. There was a great killing smog in a confined industrial valley at Liège in 1930, and a comparable peak in death rate though in a much smaller population.

It is remarkable that similarly enclosed valley settlements in South Wales and the north of England have not recorded disasters on this scale. The 1952 smog, we have suggested, may have been the last of its type. The Clean Air Acts have been given a great deal of credit for the reduction in air pollution in our cities and, while they have become effective at the same time as office and factory heating and even domestic heating has largely changed over to oil, gas or electric heating systems, there is no doubt of the reduction in urban air pollution generally. There are exceptions, in particular areas, for example, where automobile and other internal combustion engine exhausts remain a serious problem or have even increased. If external pollution and even internal pollution from open coal fires are really crucial factors in bronchitis, there ought to be a spontaneous reduction in illness and deaths from that cause within a few years. This will be all to the good but, unfortunately for analysis of the causes of the disease, there are probably other interacting factors, as has already been suggested. Some further light on such possible interactions comes from the next detailed study.

In our second study, of Leeds by John Girt, the scale of study is changed to that of a single city, and the phenomenon analysed is here morbidity or illness, not mortality.[15] For reasons of economy

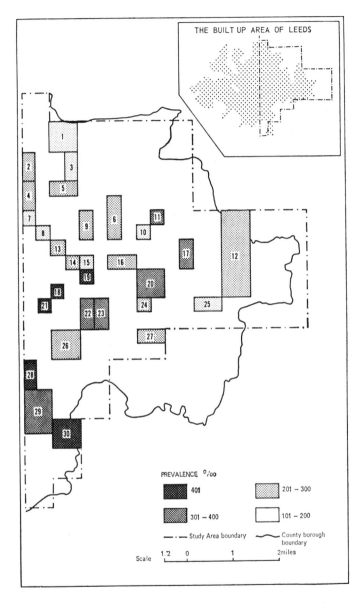

THE BUILT UP AREA OF LEEDS

PREVALENCE °/oo

	401		201 – 300
	301 – 400		101 – 200

– · – Study Area boundary   County borough boundary

Scale 1·2 0   1   2miles

Figure 53. Sample quadrats shaded for degrees of prevalence of simple chronic bronchitis in adult females. (Source: Girt, J. L. 'Simple chronic bronchitis and urban ecological structure', in McGlashan, N. D. [ed]. *Medical geography: techniques and field studies*, Methuen/University Paperbacks, 1972, Fig 16.2, p 216.)

his study was restricted to simple chronic bronchitis in adult females, and sample 'quadrats' were drawn from the eastern half of the city, though he did consider the city as a whole. The methods used in this study are of general geographical interest, so they will be discussed in more detail than most material cited in this book.

Girt began by selecting sample quadrats of varying areas, larger in area in the less populated parts of the city. In each quadrat a sample of twenty randomly selected adult females was interviewed by means of a questionnaire about symptoms of simple chronic bronchitis (without regard to the respondent's recourse or non-recourse to medical opinion or treatment), smoking habits, occupation and residential history. Prevalence

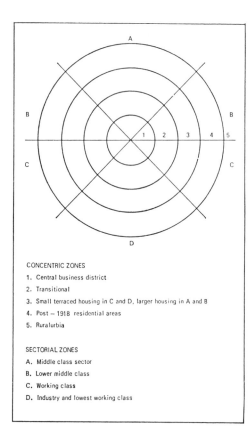

CONCENTRIC ZONES

1. Central business district
2. Transitional
3. Small terraced housing in C and D, larger housing in A and B
4. Post – 1918 residential areas
5. Ruralurbia

SECTORIAL ZONES

A. Middle class sector
B. Lower middle class
C. Working class
D. Industry and lowest working class

Figure 54. The ecological structure of a British city as applied to Leeds. (Source: as Figure 53, Girt, Fig 16.1, p 215.)

rates were calculated, mapped (Figure 53) and found significant at the 5 per cent level—ie there was only a 1 in 20 chance that the differences found were not significant, using a Poisson distribution, which is often an appropriate statistical approach in this type of problem.

Girt then adjusted the particular characteristics of Leeds to suit the combined Burgess-Hoyt model of concentric zones overlaid by sectorial slices, as adapted for British cities by a sociologist, Mann, in 1965 (Figure 54). In Leeds the industrial sector is in the southern part of the city, extending to the coalfield and middle-class suburbs to the north, so the model was modified accordingly. Prevalence rates were then calculated from the sample quadrats falling in the several concentric and sectorial zones and

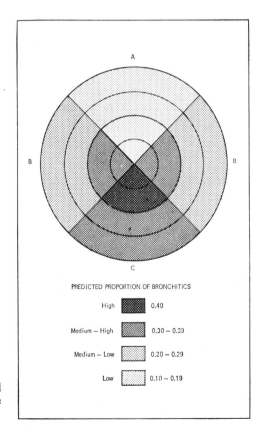

PREDICTED PROPORTION OF BRONCHITICS

High		0.40
Medium – High		0.30 – 0.39
Medium – Low		0.20 – 0.29
Low		0.10 – 0.19

Figure 55. Prevalence of simple chronic bronchitis in adult females, as predicted from the ecological model. (Source: as Figure 53, Fig 16.3, p 220.)

extrapolated to cover the whole city, as in Figure 55. Note that the B and C sectors of Figure 54 (lower-middle and working class) have been combined, since these were not found to differ significantly in bronchitis prevalence. Distance from the city centre was significantly related to decrease in bronchitis, as was sectorial or angular movement from middle-class to lower-middle/working class sectors and the industrial/lower working class sector. It is suggested that such a model of bronchitis prevalence may be capable of extension into British cities generally.

The next stage was to examine the relation of a number of possible factors to the prevalence of bronchitis by means of a series of 'regression models'; these expressed, for instance, the relation in the whole sample population between bronchitis prevalence and smoking expressed as the number of women smoking multiplied by the number of years they had smoked. This general tendency to have bronchitis was then used to simulate the bronchitis prevalence rate in each sample quadrat, by assuming that smoking-linked bronchitis was simply dispersed randomly among the whole sample population, and calculating the expected prevalence for each sample quadrat. The expected prevalence (from the simulation) could then be compared with the actual prevalence as revealed by the sample survey, quadrat by quadrat. Smoking revealed a rather unexpected result, showing much more variation according to sectors, and a greater relation to socio-economic groups, than was anticipated.

This comparison of simulated (expected) prevalence by quadrats, with actual prevalence revealed by the sample data, was carried out in turn for air pollution, overcrowding, environmental conditions (notably damp housing), and type of occupation, as well as smoking. Air pollution in the external environment did not prove significant in relation to the sample quadrat data, though Girt stresses that it might be related to the later stages of the disease more than to the simple chronic bronchitis he concentrated on for economy's sake. (Internal pollution, such as that from open fires, was not examined.) Present living conditions, of overcrowding and dampness, did not produce a close relation between the simulated and the observed prevalence, but past living conditions of overcrowding and damp housing did reveal significant relations. A final model combined the effects of past and present living conditions, and past environmental conditions and smoking, and this produced a very close resemblance to the observed conditions.

John Girt's work seems to call urgently for extension beyond Leeds to other cities, and to regional comparisons, and beyond simple chronic bronchitis, our stage 1 of the disease, to stage 2, chronic mucopurulent bronchitis, and stage 3, chronic obstructive bronchitis—and perhaps to emphysema. Meanwhile it is possible, as he himself has suggested, to read a general map like Howe's between the lines, as it were, and to envisage that parts of cities, and parts of high-bronchitis regions are largely responsible for the darker shadings of Figures 50 and 51. These parts are areas of urban stress, of poor housing and much unemployment, in which past poor and damp housing is still exacting a price, and in which, rather surprisingly, social differences in smoking habits (themselves doubtless related to economic and stress factors) play a significant part in accentuating the burden of bronchitis, the English disease.

Conclusion

I suggested in the introduction to this chapter that the two apparently non-parasitic diseases on present knowledge might form a less cohesive picture than would the infections. I think that this is true. At the same time there is something of a pattern emerging, at least in relation to the examples studied. Both of the diseases discussed are at present receiving some attention from the viewpoint that infections may be at least partially responsible. Some cancers may be associated with viruses and Burkitt's tumour with malaria. Apart from the cancers discussed in the chapter as susceptible to geographical analysis, there is growing suspicion that a small proportion of hosts of the Epstein-Barr virus, affecting the lymphatic system and causing the 'glandular fever' of popular terminology, may later suffer from cancer of the lymphatic system. There is laboratory evidence from animal experiments, but as with other cancers—think of lung cancer and smoking—it is obviously difficult to secure experimental evidence from human beings. Cancer of the cervix uteri, again, may be triggered off by infections of the genital area; the herpes virus is under suspicion here after long being regarded as normally commensal, except when erupting as 'cold sores' when the host is under attack from another parasite, such as the cold virus or malaria.

Of the 80 per cent of cancers regarded as environmental in origin, much the largest proportion are probably caused by air pollutants, self-imposed like cigarette smoke, community-made like domestic and industrial smoke, or occupational like mesothelioma, in which the cancer arises from asbestos particles.

Bronchitis seems to be primarily associated with lung irritants, usually products of our man-made environment, by prolonged rather than casual contact; but infections may attack the insulted tissues, causing much of the severe illness associated with bronchitis. This pattern should not be exaggerated: we should not be tempted to say, with a character in a play by Christopher Hampton, that one would rather that a hypothesis had form than that it should be right. For example, windy raw climates might also play a part.

My selection of diseases for this chapter has not included discussion of avoidable or premature breakdown of the cardio-vascular systems (the heart and circulation), though some spatial patterns can be observed and some relations with hard and soft water, for instance, have been debated. (The reader interested in having access to a bench-mark survey should refer to Howe and Loraine.[16]) Despite these qualifications, however, the chapter may reinforce the world view of man in relation to environmental risks, including infections and other hazards, many of which seem to be ultimately self-imposed either at individual or at community level; to that extent they are social rather than strictly environmental—or related to social rather than physical or biological environment.

CHAPTER SIX

The Geography of Hunger

Definitions

Undernutrition follows from lack of sufficient quantities of food—from hunger, in fact. It contrasts with *malnutrition*, a term that has become familiar to most people over the last 30 years or so, implying an imbalance in nutrition rather than a lack of quantity. Of course many undernourished people also suffer from malnutrition. *Overnutrition* is excess of quantity of food consumed; this surely exists in several, perhaps many, developed countries as a public-health problem (in contrast to individual cases of neurotic depraved overeating or abnormal metabolism causing obesity). An appreciable proportion, especially of males, suffer from overnutrition in the average pub or football crowd or even disco in Britain, Australia or the US, and in several western societies there is much public preoccupation with slimming in both sexes. Intuitively one tends to relate this to a combination of affluence and sedentary living, in which the manual effort has been largely removed from much work in factories, workshops and homes, as well as farms. For example, the US and the Canadian armed forces, among others, have had to adopt specific measures to control incipient or actual obesity, mainly due to overnutrition, among its (predominantly male) personnel.

The same or an overlapping group of developed countries experience a good deal of specific overnutrition in which an otherwise adequate diet is put out of balance by over-consumption of some specific element. Diseases of more or less voluntary over-consumption include, for instance, nutritional ill-balance associated with high consumption of alcohol. At the extreme alcoholism may be a serious public-health problem, as in eighteenth-century Britain, locally in Scotland still, and in some regions of modern France.[1] Specific overnutrition may contribute to, even cause, obesity and consequent problems of heart disease and circulatory disorders. These general remarks apart, such nutritional excesses of developed countries (and of many individuals in developing countries) will not be considered in this book.

Protein-calorie malnutrition can be defined as a range of pathological conditions arising from simultaneous deficiency of protein and calories and commonly associated with infections. It occurs most frequently in infants and young children.

Kwashiorkor is a protein deficiency, mainly of children on weaning. The essential factor is deficiency of amino-acids necessary for protein synthesis, with deficiency of calories as a usual contributory factor, and often infection as a precipitating one. Failure of growth, wasting, apathy and misery are among the symptoms, and in survivors crippling sequelae may be lifelong.[2]

Nutritional marasmus is a condition of muscle wasting and loss of subcutaneous fat, due largely to a form of protein-calorie malnutrition and common in infants in developing countries. Infections often seem to play an important part in producing marasmus, and it seems to be associated with late infancy, say 6–12 months, and with shanty towns etc in Third World cities, whereas kwashiorkor is seen more in toddlers of 1–2 years and in rural areas.

Undernutrition is very often associated with malnutrition in its more widespread and, on a world view, more serious form than the specific overnutritions just discussed—that is, where malnutrition arises from lack of particular constituents or ingredients such as vitamins, proteins, minerals or less commonly fats and carbohydrates. Overall sufficiency of diet is usually measured in calories, which measure the energy or fuel value of food as compared, say, with its tissue-building function, in which proteins are important.

The close connection between overall lack of food and malnutrition has been expressed in relation to remedial or preventive diets as follows: 'Look after the calories and the vitamins look after themselves.' This is true of very many reasonably mixed diets, otherwise malnutrition would be an almost world-wide problem in most socio-economic groups in most countries; and in many diets the dictum could almost be made to apply to the proteins. The protein content of most staple cereals, for instance, is such that if we look after the calories, the proteins will look after themselves. Take the protein content of rice and millet: while less than that of wheat on modern assays, rice is more readily assimilated, and but for this fact malnutrition in the rice plains of Asia would be a far more serious problem even than it is at present; several millets, again, while a low status food in many areas, possess useful protein and minerals.

The exceptions to this dictum, in relation to both vitamins and protein, make for important diseases of malnutrition. For instance, to follow up rice diets, the diets among the poorer groups of the Mahanadi-Krishna delta in eastern India not only rely too much on rice, but it is also traditionally highly milled; the milling removes the vitamin B content of the outer part of the rice grain and, before preventive measures were taken, used to leave a proportion of the population subject to the serious neural symptoms of beri-beri and to avitaminosis.

Famine or epidemic undernutrition: some case studies

The great famine in Ireland of 1845–51 was triggered off by a fungus disease of potatoes caused by *Phyophthora infestans*, brought in from America. It was favoured by the very cool and wet summers of 1845–47, and accompanied by an epidemic of louse-borne typhus and relapsing fever—'famine fever'—among stressed survivors, many of whom had become refugees. There followed a main wave of emigration, from many parts of Ireland, and from the north-west Highlands of Scotland, which had been almost as severely affected by the famine, and perhaps rather better served in famine relief. This wave of emigration turned into a stream of people leaving both areas (continuing to the present day), and halving the population of Ireland from its peak of about 8 million in the early 1840s. The famine was a complex phenomenon, and should not be regarded as simply the result of the wet years, the fungus, or for that matter patterns of landlordism and exploitation; it was also due to excessively small holdings and continuous growing of potatoes, especially in the regions of lasting difficulty in the west, and of landless labour and pauperism in every period of stress. The causes were multiple and interacting. Yet the events are of some relevance to our own time, for they did succeed a sort of population explosion, itself complex in origins.[3]

The potato disease followed a period of marked population increase, almost comparable to the population increase in many underdeveloped countries today. Some historians have suggested that a large part was played by smallpox vaccinations, which were widely disseminated following Jenner's experiments of 1796. The reduction in child mortality in particular, it is suggested, was crucial in causing this earlier population explosion in Ireland and similar areas, though historical demographers are not convinced, at least on existing evidence.

The population explosion was made possible, in a sense, by the introduction of the potato, which brought a new and very high yielding staple source of belly-filling starchy food to areas like western Ireland, complementing and reducing the relative importance of hardy cereals like oats, arctic barley and rye. In good times the substantial vitamin C content of potatoes made it a good staple food, and many contemporary accounts of Ireland before the famine comment favourably on the appearance and liveliness of people in the countryside. There was, no doubt, population pressure even with the potato. But without the potato, when the blight brought widespread failure of the crop in several successive years, the population pressure became insupportable, and in the absence of adequate relief measure the Malthusian check of deaths from famine reaped its grim harvest. Not all areas, and not all socio-economic groups in the population, were equally vulnerable, and a case can be argued that the famine, though triggered off by a series of wet years encouraging a fungus disease of potatoes, was yet a man-made rather than a natural disaster.[4]

More recently something of the same combination occurred in the great famine in the Ukraine and south-western Russia in the years 1919–21, in which several million people died. There was a sequence of climatic vagaries, this time a series of drought years, causing widespread failure of the wheat crop. But the famine could no doubt have been prevented, or at least prevented from being a major catastrophe, had it not been for a number of man-made elements in the disaster. Those early years following the Russian Revolution of 1917 were times of much chaos and civil war, and the conditions were much too disorganized and disturbed to permit the smooth flow of the massive amounts of food needed to counteract the famine within the USSR.

There were massive international relief efforts, by Herbert Hoover's American Relief Commission, by Quaker and other religious groups, and by appeals headed by the Norwegian polar explorer Nansen; but relations between the still insecure revolutionary government and potentially subversive foreigners were naturally uneasy. All efforts failed to avert the catastrophe, and, as often happens, famine was followed by epidemics, including typhus (as in Ireland in 1845–47), adding to the mortality.

We can link the Russian famine of 1919–21 also with mid-latitude climates of moderately low rainfalls of high variability from year to year. These will support cereal crops in a good year but not in a poor one, and a sequence of poor years may mean hardship, loss of land, and perhaps migration to the city for capitalist farmers. The famine tracts, looking at history and geography together, are those parts of the world where moderate to low and variable rainfall is combined with what is substantially subsistence farming, whether peasant or tribal. Areas of comparable climate, but with cash rather than subsistence farming for stock or cereals (parts of Australia, for instance), do not suffer famines, though they may have periods of severe stress during series of successive drought years—or indeed in more purely man-made financial blizzards. Of course famine relief measures are possible, but the famine tracts remain vulnerable.

The Bengal famine of 1943–44 occurred in a normally humid climate, and was basically a rice famine, affecting people very much used to the easily assimilable rice; once weakened by famine, they were in real difficulties in turning to other diets, though a starving man is not a food faddist. The famine had something of the tragic combination of natural and man-made disaster of the post-revolution famine in Russia. There was a local hurricane and a flood disaster south of Calcutta in October 1942, and in the next year some crop failure because of disease affecting the rice plants. The war loomed large. The Japanese were on the eastern borders of Bengal, which was a major base of Allied defensive power, where attacking forces were being built up for the reinvasion of Burma. Wartime secrecy and censorship prevailed.

This is a semi-aquatic deltaic environment, poor in roads and railways, and very dependent on western-type barges and even more on 'country' boats in every village and on every creek and deltaic distributary. In fear of Japanese invasion many country boats had been commandeered, and others sunk or destroyed, in order to deny them to invading forces. Local famine broke out, normal communications—exaggerated rumour apart—did not operate, and normal famine relief measures were not applied. Panic buying and hoarding followed, and inevitably buying and hoarding by speculators and profiteers. Soon the famine spread further than it need have done. Thousands of people left their villages and flocked to the towns and cities, especially Calcutta, which already had enough problems of its own and was unable to cope with the influx, despite many piecemeal efforts by the city authorities, and others. I recall visiting the home of a Muslim high court judge, and found his garden full of thatch and bamboo huts occupied by a score of refugees whom he was feeding and succouring. Hundreds of people died in the Calcutta streets daily, and thousands more in the villages or on the roads.

Disease followed, as in the refugee movements accompanying the Bangladesh war of independence in 1972, for the Bengal delta is the world endemic home of cholera. Terrible damage had been done, millions of lives lost, and millions more had been irreparably scarred by physical and mental damage, before effective relief measures began. The Viceroy, Lord Wavell, eventually got to know of the enormous scale of the disaster, and insisted on the diversion of troops and supplies to deal with famine relief; Westminster eventually also was apprised of the true scale of the catastrophe and the wartime security and censorship veils were torn away. The procurement of rice was taken over by the government, which recruited prominent men from the trade, and effective rationing and the flow to needy areas were organized at last, along with improvised strategic storage depots. (Alas, in the Bengal climate some of these suffered much destruction of the rice by rotting, fungus etc!) Not least, a later world famous Bengali physicist and statistician, P. C. Mahalanobis, designed a new system of sampling crops by cutting sample plots to improve forecasting of harvest yields for the future. So some forward thinking at least emerged from a terrible disaster, a most terrible blot on the closing years of the British raj in India.

Compared with the historical examples, our basis of assessment has become more quantitative. This does not mean that all problems of assessment have been solved, but at least some rough and ready numbers are in use. In Figure 57 a figure of 2,000 calories per day has been taken as a watershed between areas with adequate 'daily bread' and those without. There are problems of interpretation. Colder climates make more demands on the body in maintaining heat in the absence of much artificial heating of buildings, or adequate clothing. Manual work is much more demanding than sedentary work in respect of calorific needs from one's diet. But there is increasing empirical evidence from widely contrasting areas that the 2,000 calorie mark serves as a rough indicator of the watershed between sufficiency and hunger.

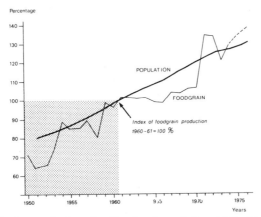

Figure 56. India, graph of trends of food and population, 1949–76. (Source: Open University. 'The population explosion, an interdisciplinary "approach"', in *Understanding Society* course, Fig 33.3, p 42.)

134

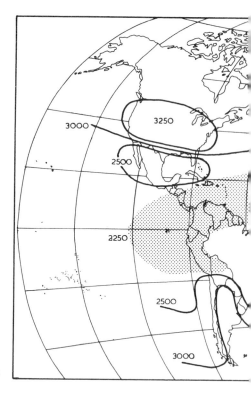

Figure 57. World map showing
average diet intake: shaded area
shows less than 2,000 calories.
(Source: updated from Linton
D. L. 'The geography of energy',
Geography, 50, 1965, 197–228.)

Apart from qualifications (below) about simplistic interpreta-
tions of the map it should be noted that a distinguished student of
population and development, Colin Clark, with a good deal of
Third World experience, does not believe that half or two-thirds of
the world's population suffer from malnutrition and actual
hunger, as claimed by the World Food and Agricultural
Organization as long ago as 1950; this is because he thinks that
the standards by which these are defined are based on western
diets, which in fact often produce overnutrition, as we have
noted.[5] However, 2,000 calories a day does seem a realistic
minimum average standard for countries where many people are
engaged in agriculture; there are slack seasons, usually in hot dry
weather, when smaller food intakes may suffice, but it remains
true that for many families food shortage increases through the
dry season, and it is very short when the rains come and hard

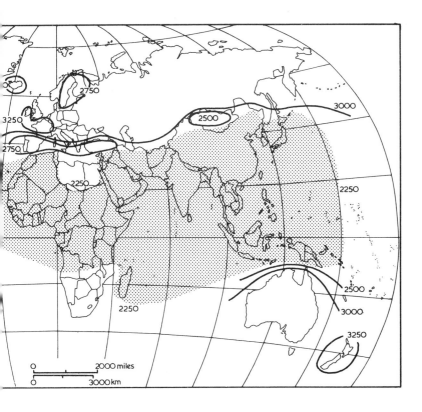

work has to be done. My view is that the figure is at least worthy
of study in a cautious way.

Most of the hungry countries fall within the Third World,
mainly in the tropics, but not all tropical countries are below the
2,000 calorie mark—note Central America on Figure 57 and
much of Africa south of the equator. Moreover the generalization
of the map is extreme, as it must be using data by nation-states;
there are certainly substantial pockets of very well fed people in
inter-tropical Africa, for instance, some following traditional
ways, some the modern life style. (Some of the latter doubtless
suffering from overnutrition, including specific overnutritions
such as alcohol poisoning!) The average by countries, too, con-
ceals differences by socio-economic strata. Within the population
of many, perhaps all, countries there are particularly vulnerable
groups of economically disadvantaged people, such as

unemployed landless labourers in rural India or frequently
unemployed day labourers in the towns and cities throughout
the Third World. These underprivileged groups represent
considerable minorities who are liable to be well below the
2,000 calorie mark not only in countries below that figure but
in many with higher values. There are tracts of chronic undernutrition though there are good years and bad, as we see from
Figure 56.

As so often remedies seem to lie in the complex and difficult,
but not impossible, operation we simplify as development
programmes.

Famine areas

Periodic famines occur rather like epidemics. Figures 58 and 59
attempt to show first what one might call traditional famine tracts,
which lie mainly in areas of low to moderate rainfall with low
reliability (or high variability, to employ the usual statistical term
with recognized methods of calculation). Wide tracts of the more
arid areas of the Old World have for much of human history been
occupied by nomadic herders; while drought and famine may
strike, and their herds be decimated month by month or even
week by week until the stock are almost extinct, the nomads are
by definition mobile, used to moving out from the parched graz-
ings in search of greener lands. Sometimes they have swept out as
marauders or conquerors, as in the recurrent waves of herder-
cavalrymen moving outwards from Central Asia. Sometimes they
move out more quietly, in smaller groups, to make their living as
best they can, usually with the idea of returning to their herds and
pastures as soon as conditions permit. The Tuareg of the Saharan
margins, for instance, moved out in just this way during the recent
drought years in the Sahel area of Africa, and many have now
moved back following renewed rains.

More numerous and more affected by drought and famine are
sedentary cultivators, who in times of hardship may find that they
had to contend with the outward-moving nomads as well as the
harshness of nature. Farming towards the climatic margins of
agriculture, they are used to gambling on the chances of the
weather suiting their staple crops even more than farmers

everywhere, and a series of drought years may reduce them to real extremity, especially if there are economic millstones in the way of debt to face, as well as natural hazards. The traditional famine tracts of Figures 58 and 59 lie mainly in such regions: in the areas on the margins of the Old World deserts in Africa north and south of the Sahara, right across the Middle East and into Central Asia and north-western China, in parts of India, and in north-eastern Brazil. While some of these areas have moderate rainfall, they also have high variability.

While there are many human factors in famine, Figures 58 and 59 enable us to view famine and precipitation or rainfall from two aspects: (a) mean annual precipitation and (b) annual variability of rainfall—high variability is simply low reliability. Many, though not all, famines occur in years of low rainfall (occasionally of excess rainfall) in areas where the mean annual precipitation is marginal to the requirements of particular food crops, especially staple cereals. While detailed analysis would require careful analysis of the moisture needs of the individual crop—or even individual variety—through the growing season, we may think of the following marginal mean annual rainfall as marginal for the crops noted: rice 40in (100cm); wheat 15in (38cm); and drought-resistant millets (of several genera and species) 10in (25 cm). Reading Figures 58 and 59 together, we see risk of famine if there is a coincidence of (a) marginal rainfall for the staple food crop, (b) high variability of rainfall (or low reliability) and (c) a dominance of subsistence rather than developed capitalist, mixed-economy or communist farming. Thus of the areas numbered on the maps, and referred to in the text, area 1 is an area of wheat farming in a mixed economy, so drought years or series of drought years are marked by hardship rather than famine; similarly in areas 3, 4, 5, 12, 13 and 14, though older readers will recall near-famine conditions reported from the Dust Bowl area of the USA in the 1930s, and we earlier noted the terrible concatenation of circumstances in south-western Russia in 1919–21. Area 2 is an example of famine in a humid tract of normally reliable rainfall—the potato famine areas of Ireland and Scotland discussed earlier. Area 2 is again an example of a convergence of adverse factors, as is area 8 in Bengal, which saw the famine of

138

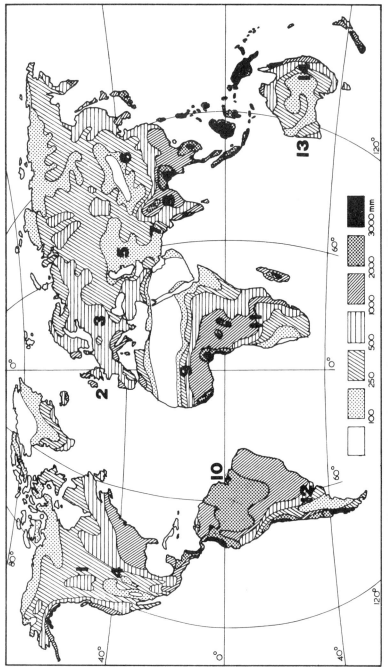

Figure 58. Mean annual precipitation. (Source: *Pergamon World Atlas*, 1968.)

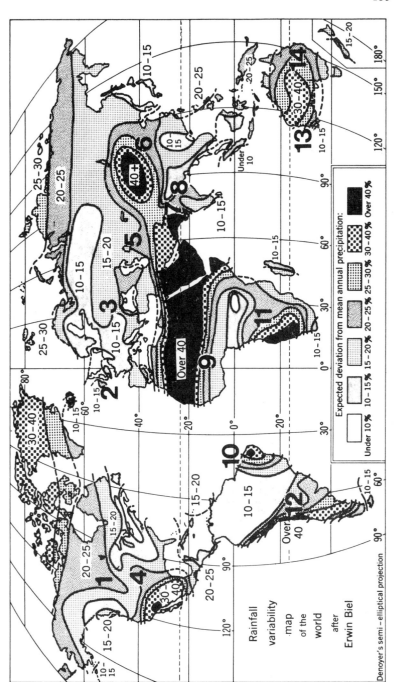

Figure 59. Variability of rainfall. (Source: Biel, E. and American Geographical Society, in Strahler A. N. *Physical Geography*, 1961, Fig 13.9, p 199.)

1943–44 noted above; just to the north-west lies Bihar, which has seen more than one near-famine or controlled famine since Indian independence. This is an example of a quite rainy area where famine has occurred because moderate variability brings the rainfall too low for rice cultivation in drought years; farther west this occurs also in maize-growing areas, while area 10 in Brazil has seen many famines, near-famines or in recent years controlled famines in a mainly maize-growing tract in the north-east. Area 7 lies in the main area of low to moderate precipitation and rather high variability in India, where many famines, controlled in recent years, have occurred in both wheat and millet-growing areas, while area 6 indicates analogous conditions in China. Area 9 indicates the Sahel tract south of the Sahara, which saw several years of drought, loss of cattle and famine in the early 1970s, accentuated by rising population; and area 11 is the analogue area in southern Africa in which subsistence farmers are liable to famine, more or less controlled in recent years, whereas capitalist farmers are liable to years of hardship and financial loss, possibly even loss of their land in a run of dry years.

In all these regions it is the peasant farmer who is liable to be the victim of famine. A cash farmer, such as the Australian stock owner, may encounter harsh financial times, and may even have to leave the land, but he does not experience famine; so areas of comparable climate in developed areas such as North America, southern Latin America, white South Africa, Australia, New Zealand, and, in recent decades, the USSR, also experience difficulty and hardship but not outright famine. North-eastern Brazil, a recurrently famine-stricken tract in recent centuries, is different from the other areas mentioned: whereas all the rest are towards the margins of grain farming of even quite drought-resistant crops, the staple grain crop of north-eastern Brazil is maize, which needs moderate to high summer rainfall.

This reminds us that, as well as the familiar famine tracts on the very margins of sown land, there are areas on the climatic margins of more moisture-demanding crops, such as maize, rice, or even rain-forest root crops like cassava and yams. The present population explosion may be increasing the threat of famine in such areas, locally at least, by producing population pressure on resources that is likely to be harmful to both people and environment. Such population pressure could be avoided if population increase is accompanied, for instance, by changes in technology or economic diversification. One symptom of such locally increasing population pressure is famine in drought years, flood years, or years of irregular patterns of precipitation—in India, for instance, in rain-fed maize tracts of moderate mean annual rainfalls in the middle Ganga plains, and in normally wetter rice tracts farther east in eastern Uttar Pradesh and northern Bihar.

Even areas of usually reliable rainfall—moderate or high rainfalls which are of moderate to high reliability—may have many undernourished people. Commonly undernourishment is ever present, endemic rather than epidemic, and seemingly clear evidence of population pressure: for instance, in West Bengal, where it is particularly apparent among economically vulnerable groups like landless labourers. Much of the alarm about the population explosion arises from fears that this form of constantly sapping undernutrition may be very widespread, and spreading. It is associated with protein-calorie malnutrition, including the impact of infectious disease. The maxim noted earlier about calories and vitamins may be turned about: chronically meagre quantities of mainly starchy food almost as axiomatically lead to malnutrition, notably protein malnutrition. The axiom overstates somewhat, for it is necessary to allow for the substantial proportions and assimilability of protein in the starchy food, like those noted earlier for rice, and adult needs for tissue maintenance are normally less than those of growing children. On the other hand, the head of the household is apt to get the lion's share, including any protein foods available, in most cultures.

Protein

The man in the street in recent decades is increasingly aware of the need for protein for growth and tissue maintenance. Here we concentrate on protein as a problem of the underdeveloped world, drawing largely on United Nations Publications.[6]

The word protein was coined in 1838 for what was then regarded as the proto—first or primary—constituent of plant and animal bodies or material, and though its usage now differs from the original one, the fundamental importance of protein remains, for, along with the 80 per cent of water, its 20 per cent makes up the bulk of the human body. All proteins contain carbon, hydrogen, oxygen and the key constituent nitrogen; most contain sulphur and many contain such other elements as phosphorus, iron, iodine and copper. There are many different proteins, arising from permutations in combination among about twenty-eight amino-acids (other amino-acids being 'free' amino-acids). The protein-forming amino-acids include both basic amino groups (of nitrogen and hydrogen molecules, usually as NH_2) and acid carboxyl groups (of molecules of carbon, oxygen and hydrogen, usually as COOH), which are linked by rings of carbon molecules of various shapes and by further carbon-hydrogen molecule combinations, so that the 'building blocks' are assembled in permutations to form the vast range of different proteins.

The process of digestion breaks down proteins in food into the constituent amino-acids, and reassembles the amino-acids into proteins needed for growth, tissue replacement etc. The body can synthesize some amino-acids, but cannot synthesize the 'essential amino-acids'; these are 'essential' in the sense that they must and can come only from the diet. Vegetable protein often lacks some essential amino-acids, even plants rich in protein; animal protein, in contrast, stands at the end of a process of digestion analogous to that in man, and is commonly more complete. Plant foods, in other words, vary widely in the degree to which they approach the combination of amino-acids required to meet human protein needs, and in the digestibility of the vegetable protein, whereas animal protein tends to be both more digestible and of higher quality in the sense of biological value to the human organism. In a nutritionist's technical term they tend to have higher net protein utilization.

In fact a few particular foods rich in animal protein, such as eggs, human milk and cows' milk, seem to approach as closely as possible at present to the idea of a 'reference protein' against which other, perhaps new, forms of protein food can be measured—for instance, the synthetic protein produced by yeasts from petroleum wastes, or combinations of vegetable foods manufactured in developing countries to provide protein-rich foods without dependence on imported milk etc.

Of the vegetable foods, those rich in assimilable protein include pulses (peas, beans etc), oilseeds, certain cereals (notably rice and millets, which are superior in net protein utilization to wheat, though not necessarily in protein content, weight for weight) and some leafy vegetables like amaranth and spinach. (Spinach is also rich in iron but apparently not in a very assimilable form.) At the other end of the scale the starchy tropical root-crops like cassava (tapioca, after processing to remove hydrogen cyanide from the tuber), yams and sweet potato, and also the banana, all offer to man very poor and poorly utilized protein.

Vegetable sources provide about 70 per cent of the world's protein food, including about 50 per cent of the world protein from cereals; some 12 per cent from pulses, oilseeds and nuts; about 4 per cent from tropical tubers etc; and about 4 per cent from other vegetables and fruit. Of the 32 per cent of world protein from animal sources, meat and poultry provide some 15 per cent, milk 11 per cent, fish 4 per cent and eggs 2 per cent. The poor and poorly utilized protein content of the tropical root-crops raises particular difficulties, not so much for adults as for children, who are physically incapable of consuming large enough quantities of these staple foods, even if they are available to them, to make up the heavy needs of protein in relation to their body weight that are characteristic of growing children. It is in relation to problems like these that the world map of protein, vitamin and mineral deficiencies should be considered (Figure 62), along with the very strong traditions of what foods are suitable for children, especially sick children, the equally strong tendency to give preference in foods considered most nourishing to the breadwinner, and so on. Some of the results in undernutrition and particularly in malnutrition will now be outlined.

Protein-calorie malnutrition is preferred by some authorities to the term protein-calorie deficiency. Aykroyd for one prefers the former as a broader term, allowing for malnutrition in individuals where dietary intake may include just enough of both proteins and calories but in whom symptoms are precipitated by other factors, particularly bacterial and viral infections. It particularly affects infants and young children, with effects ranging from extreme bodily wasting to kwashiorkor. Protein malnutrition does occur in adults, and may be increasing as an endemic feature of people under population pressure, as suggested above. It is difficult to be clear about malnutritions over the last few decades because of changing ideas about terminology, but it does seem that protein-calorie malnutrition can occur as a kind of epidemic among populations under stress. One example used to occur among the streams of mainly male migrant labourers who used to walk long distances from the former Ruanda-Urundi, in the then Belgian Congo, for agricultural work in Uganda. In Africa, a continent of movement of people, there must be many such occurrences. It must occur after natural or man-made disasters—hurricanes and floods, earthquakes and volcanic eruptions, war and refugee movements. The enormous streams of people moving from East Pakistan to West Bengal before the war that brought independence to Bangladesh in 1972 were subject, as such movements often are, to epidemics of infectious disease—in that case of cholera and smallpox. Apart from the immediate toll of deaths, there is often lasting damage to the body's growth mechanisms, possibly to the bone-marrow, whose vital functions lie in producing the blood cells, but not apparently to the immune mechanisms. Clearly the implications are particularly serious for infants and children.

Kwashiorkor, as noted earlier, is the usual term for protein malnutrition of weanlings. The word comes from the Ga dialect of coastal Ghana and means 'first-second', implying the disease of the first child when the second follows too closely. Early writers about kwashiorkor translated the term as meaning 'the red boy', though with the implication of 'deprived child' or 'supplanted child'. A reddish tinge in normally black hair and skin is a common external symptom of this malnutrition, and some others, and came to be associated with deprivation, particularly when a child was displaced from breast feeding by a new baby regarded as born too soon after his elder sibling by the standard of local customs and taboos. Traditionally breast feeding commonly continues for the first few years of a child's life, whereas such a displaced child is often weaned on to an excessively starchy diet, so causing the malnutrition, for unfortunately several of the staple starchy foods used in tropical Africa are particularly poor in protein. This is especially true of cassava (tapioca), maize and—much more locally—bananas.

Figure 60 is a map of known occurrence of kwashiorkor as a significant public-health problem in the mid-1950s. The association with underdeveloped tropical countries is partly because a questionnaire, upon which the plotting was based, was applied only in tropical and sub-tropical countries; but fading out towards their margins is clear, as is the association with underdevelopment. This is true even though countries with better medical facilities are more likely to report cases than countries with very few such services; note, for instance, the frequency of records from South Africa. Indeed Cicely Williams, who introduced the name kwashiorkor into literature, suggested that a map of this type is really a map of paediatricians.

Nevertheless the map shows the importance of the disease in Africa and under conditions of much higher population densities in India; it occurs in Djakarta, then a city almost overwhelmed by the post-independence problems, not the least of which was an enormous influx from overpopulated rural Java into peri-urban shanty towns, and yet the syndrome is also recorded from the relative prosperity of Singapore and Malaysia and not necessarily only in extremely underprivileged groups. While the relation with amino-acids deficiency, especially on weaning, may be clear, the ecological relations are clearly diverse, though both poverty and ignorance will almost always be involved and just occasionally ignorance even combined with relative prosperity. Mapping is not sufficiently sensitive to justify causal analysis but, combining the literature and correspondence with doctors all over the tropics a few years ago, the writer can suggest some causal factors, though some are matters of opinion.

In Europe, apart from wartime siege conditions—for instance, in Budapest—occurrence seems to be quite exceptional and due to dietary ignorance, mistaken tradition or fads. For example, in Greece a diet of ricewater and rice soup is taken after diarrhoea.

From the Middle East there were reports of kwashiorkor from Israel soon after the formation of the state, especially in poor Arab children, often breast-fed but with inadequate lactation from a poorly fed mother, inadequate family use of milk and dairy products or eggs, and poor diets of cornflour, vegetable soup and bread. Similarly in vulnerable groups in Egypt the normal weaning diet seems to include a very little milk and some boiled beans or lentils, but infants with kwashiorkor were fed largely on cereal water; 'summer diarrhoea' seems to be a precipitating factor. Elsewhere in the Middle East incidence seems to be sporadic. Sorghum millet was thought not to lead to the syndrome.

Moving into north-west Africa there was kwashiorkor in poor Muslim labourers' families living in one-room hovels, with prolonged lactation—perhaps too long and likely to be interrupted by another pregnancy. Supplementary or weaning diet was largely the semolina-like cous-cous. In West Africa as a whole kwashiorkor seemed to be recorded in urban rather than rural communities. In the drier northern belt this was true, though the syndrome was thought to be unusual but associated with poor urban diets. The rural problem was much more severe seasonal undernutrition in the hungry weeks and months before the harvest. In the south the traditional diet includes much more of the low-protein root-crops, and under poor urban conditions, where meat or fish are too dear to contribute much to low food budgets, even adult diets are highly starchy, and weaning is largely on to tapioca pap. Suckling for very prolonged periods, up to 5 or 6 years, was not unknown, nor was suckling by grand-mothers, aunts etc, and poor human milk was suspected as a cause in some cases. In Sudan and Eritrea nomadic communities were thought not to have much kwashiorkor, but it was known from peasants and town-dwellers, in infants weaned on to maize rather than millet or milk foods.

In Central and East Africa kwashiorkor was thought to be a disease of open plateaux rather than forest terrain, where, despite consumption of root-crops, there was a wealth of supplementary items of diet, including animal protein, to be picked up by toddlers eating caterpillars, ants etc; and it was regarded as likely to occur in the hungry period before the maize harvest or in poor urban groups divorced from unconsidered dietary supplements in the bush. A growing infant could not consume the bulk of starchy cereals needed to give it adequate vegetable protein from that source, and by tradition the protein-rich groundnut, pulse, meat, fish or sauce are thought 'too rich' for weanlings.

In South Africa kwashiorkor was not commonly recorded among poor urban Africans (Bantu and Zulu) away from traditional rural diets, but there was a disquieting increase in some rural areas, where the disease seemed to be clearly related to weaning on to maize diets. Zulu women in traditional communities are subject to taboos on the use of dairy products, thus adding to the problem.

There was little doubt of widespread occurrence of kwashiorkor in India, perhaps with slightly different groups of symptoms in the syndrome among rice-eaters and in communities using other staple cereals. It was found overwhelmingly among the poor and ignorant, occasionally among the rich and ignorant, and often with infections, especially intestinal, as precipitating factors. Findings elsewhere in South Asia were consistent with these, with urban and rural poor both affected. In Malaysia and Singapore there were occurrences among relatively prosperous groups in cities, including Chinese, and the problem seemed to be one of dietary education. Rural cases among poorer Malay families were also thought to be fairly common. The position was rather similar in Indonesia, where much larger numbers are reported from the slums of such main cities as Djakarta and Makassar, and from a wide variety of farming areas (some with rice as the staple diet, some maize, some tubers, some sago). Often dysentery and other infections were present also. Over-prolonged breast feeding was under suspicion as a factor.

In the Pacific kwashiorkor was not regarded as common, It did occur in Fiji, however, especially among poor Indian families with frequent pregnancies.

The West Indies brought no definite reports, because of doubts about the definition of what is after all a syndrome or group of symptoms rather than a specific disease, but there are certainly reports in the literature of similar protein malnutritions. Central American reports regarded some of their protein malnutritions as kwashiorkor, and the problem as one largely of education in weaning diets rather than necessarily of poverty, though

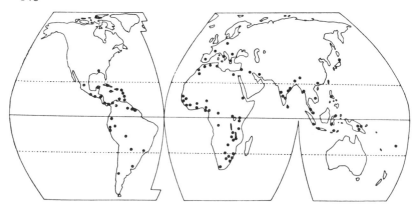

Figure 60. World map of kwashiorkor, a protein malnutrition. (Source: Learmonth, A. T. A. 'Kwashiorkor: social and geographical relationship of a malnutrition of the underdeveloped area', in 'This Changing World', *Geography*, 41, 1956, p 62.)

incidence was in comparatively underprivileged urban groups.

Kwashiorkor has been recognized in every country in South America, and it seems to be common in poor populations in many parts of the tropical areas—for instance, in poor mestizo or part-Indian farming groups, where milk is rare and weaning on to maize gruel, or on to barley gruel in highland areas, is common. The temperate countries regarded the condition as almost as rare as in Europe.

Since Figure 60 was compiled, kwashiorkor has continued to be reported almost every month in the abstracting journals, so that a dot map would cover very much of the developing world, still with a thicker concentration where health services are good enough to report the syndrome and investigate it. We must almost regard this as a nutritional disease of the poor and underprivileged in nearly all parts of the Third World. Hence Figure 61 is the best representation of the broader problem of which kwashiorkor is a part.

Remedial measures

Protein malnutrition, including kwashiorkor, can be treated, if it is not too advanced. The first reaction of local-health authorities and of international organizations was to turn to protein-rich supplements like skim-milk powder, and to introduce it into toddlers' diets in hospitals and health centres, as well as trying to

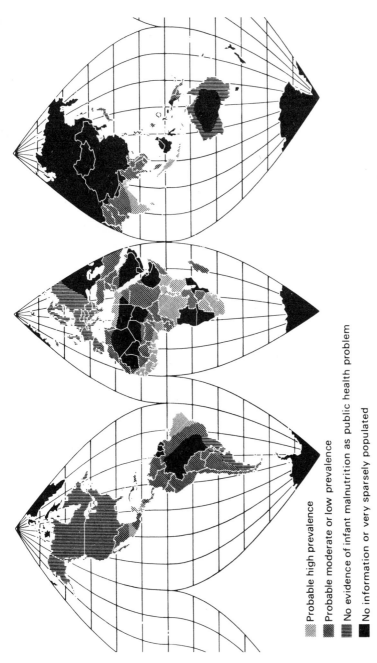

Figure 61. World map of infant malnutrition. (Source: FAO/WHO/UNICEF Protein Advisory Group. *Lives in peril: protein and the child*, World Food Problems No 12, Rome, FAO, 1970, pp 30 and 42.)

Probable high prevalence

Probable moderate or low prevalence

No evidence of infant malnutrition as public health problem

No information or very sparsely populated

ensure that it was included in their diet at home. This sort of measure is not satisfactory for various reasons. Not all skim-milk powders are suitable for infants in lieu of mother's milk, for some contain excess salt and others lack essential vitamins. The provision of such food supplements, whether from health authorities or by international aid organizations, is no doubt necessary and even possibly commendable as a temporary and palliative measure, but it is a piece of external intervention rather than something built into the local diet, and does nothing for dietary education. Worse, it is a sort of dole or charity. Moreover there is good evidence that in many tropical areas there is intolerance of lactose, the sugars contained in the dried milk powders.

Knowledge is coming forward from some areas of ways in which both these difficulties may be surmounted, if only the logistics or organizational problems can be mastered on both the technological and the educational fronts. Locally grown vegetable protein can be incorporated into diets, especially weaning diets, in quantities and with the specific amino-acids needed for protein absorption and normal growth patterns—for instance soya beans can be grown over a very wide area of the tropics, and, if they are not readily assimilable into traditional dietaries, can be processed into locally acceptable foods. In the tapioca-producing area of south-western India soya has been processed with tapioca into rice-like grains that could be widely acceptable. More recently a cereal-soya-milk combination has been manufactured by extrusion under pressure to form palatable crisp-like flakes, which have proved highly acceptable in nursery schools and as school lunches in South India. While this sort of problem will have to be tackled quite locally, in all probability, it does offer much more hopeful prospects in the long term than the temporary supply of milk powder, even where the people can take it.

At the same time the effort needed to make good the shortages of protein the world over remains immense. It is difficult to think of a more pressing world problem, especially in view of the loss of life, the misery of the victims, and the growing evidence of crippling ill-effects during the lifetime of those affected, and even on the children of women who suffered from protein malnutrition when they were themselves children. There is little doubt that technologically this problem can still be contained—for instance, by biochemical methods of protein production.[7]

Vitamin deficiencies

Other forms of malnutrition are mainly caused by lack of a specific vitamin—sometimes of course by more than one—and commonly combined with undernutrition and perhaps protein malnutrition as well (Figures 62 and 63). Again developed countries can understand the problem from their own history. Scurvy, due to lack of vitamin C, was common in seamen in the days of sail, and the ration of lemon or lime insisted on by some far-sighted captains was the origin of the American derisory name for the English as 'limeys'.

Rickets, a grave malformation of the bones, especially the large bones, in growing children, is due to lack of vitamin D from sunlight, replaceable by cod-liver oil or halibut oil and the like. It was formerly rampant in many poor areas in British cities, notably Glasgow. It almost disappeared with wartime rationing and school milk, but has recently reappeared as a significant public-health problem, particularly in Glasgow, partly among indigenous groups and partly among immigrants, particularly those from Pakistan. The end of rationing brought a decreased standard of balance in nutrition to vulnerable groups in the population. Loss of milk subsidy, the progressive cessation of school milk (except in primary schools at the time of writing), decreasing use of infant-welfare clinics—all these have played their part. Rickets is still active in some Third World countries, especially in poor Muslim groups or even some prosperous ones, where women and children in purdah may not see the sun very much, even in sunny countries. There is also a somewhat analogous disease of bone formation during pregnancy called osteomalacia, which has similar causes. Scurvy is still a significant problem in Himalayan villages in the Almora district in northern India, according to Rais Akhtar's recent doctoral thesis to Aligarh Muslim University, with vitamin A deficiency and eye disease.

In Figure 62, a world map of protein, vitamin and mineral deficiencies, the association with the underdeveloped world is clear. Considering the consequences to health, this is a depressing

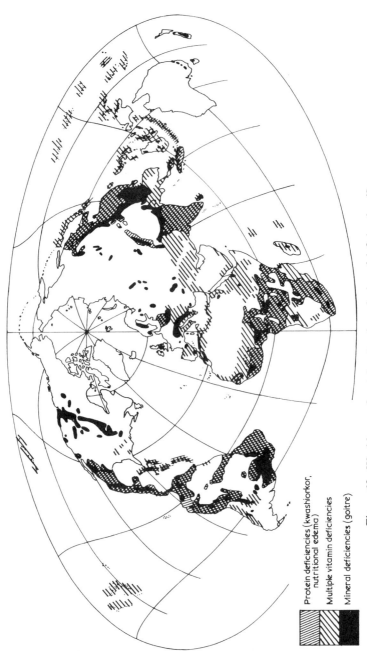

Figure 62. World map of protein, vitamin and mineral deficiencies. (Source: after May, J. M. 'World Atlas of Diseases No 9', *Geog Rev*, 43, 1953.)

Protein deficiencies (kwashiorkor, nutritional edema)

Multiple vitamin deficiencies

Mineral deficiencies (goitre)

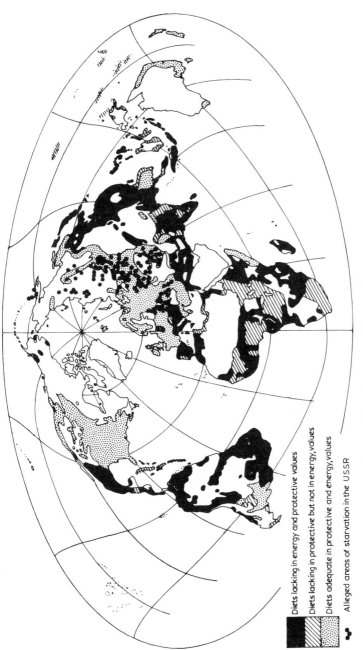

Figure 63. World map of diets. (Source: as Figure 62.)

Diets lacking in energy and protective values

Diets lacking in protective but not in energy, values

Diets adequate in protective and energy, values

Alleged areas of starvation in the USSR

map. Short-term solutions to the problem of vitamins by the distribution of vitamin tablets are relatively easy and cheap to administer, but longer-term solutions are a matter of nutritional education and sometimes of campaigns to diversify local cropping patterns with acceptable foods rich in the missing vitamins. In this the problem resembles protein malnutrition, though it is somewhat less grave, as well as easier to solve in the short term. Perhaps the most outstanding urgent vitamin deficiency to be tackled by the developing countries and international agencies is vitamin A deficiency, which causes a considerable proportion of the blindness in the developing world. This vitamin, obtainable from foods like eggs and dairy produce, and from palm oil, for example, assists the maintenance of the soft tissues, mucous membrane etc, and severe and prolonged lack of it produces ulceration and scarring of the eyes and ultimately blindness. Like other vitamin deficiencies it is readily prevented, even cured for early cases, by short-term vitamin supplements. In the long term dietary education and better diets may be more difficult.

Undernutrition and communication

Undernutrition in developed countries, again, may be thought of as almost a problem of communication, though most commonly it is linked to economic factors, to poverty and to the costs of eliminating hunger due to poverty. An example is undernutrition, commonly accompanied by malnutrition, among old people. Hunger is surely more common among poor old people than rich old people, who are able to pay for support and services even when they are alone in the world. Very lonely old people who are also poor are much more likely to go hungry or to fill their bellies with an ill-balanced diet, or in countries with cold winters to die of hypothermia on cold nights. Is it then a problem of communication? It may often be so.

An institution like the British 'Meals on Wheels' service is one type of formal and organized response to the communication problem. The improvement in communication is a directly physical one, linking the person in need to a flow of nourishing meals by suitable forms of food supply, storage and transport. This organization, of course, is only able to go into action if it has information about old people needing help. It is in respect of information about need that undernutrition among the old is so great, and often so baffling, a communication problem. No doubt it would be possible to analyse this problem geographically, but it is difficult to make actual studies.

It is easy to visualize a geographical survey of old people in an area, perhaps with some classification of their likely need for 'Meals on Wheels', for a certain period of years. Like several other symptoms of social malaise, this problem has some concentration in inner city areas; the Liverpool inner city study, for instance, showed how adults in need of free meals can be one indicator of a whole complex of deprivations.[8] Such a survey could be followed by working out an optimal or at least suboptimal pattern of supply points and transport flow. But this belongs to the nascent geography of medical care discussed in Chapter 8.

In developed countries in recent decades, the problems of under-nutrition and malnutrition are both limited, and largely concealed; so it is quite difficult to arouse, and even more to hold, the public attention on hunger as a serious world problem, even though many individuals are more or less knowledgeable and more or less critically intelligent about it. Yet historically, as we have seen, hunger was present just a few decades or a few generations ago, and it should not be impossible to make contact with the collective consciousness, and conscience, in this grave problem.

Before leaving the topic of the geography of hunger, let us turn to a deficiency that even less than the vitamin deficiencies can be described as any form of hunger. That is iodine deficiency, the main cause of goitre.

Goitre

Goitre is enlargement of the thyroid gland in the neck, the word being derived through French from the Latin *guttur*, throat. It is one of the several terms used in England for the disease at various periods; others are Derbyshire neck, struma (Latin for scrofula), and scrofula itself, though that also applies to swellings of the lymphatic system, as did king's evil (from the idea that the disease could be cured by the touch of the king). It is a matter of some significance that the popular term goitre, indicating only enlargement of the thyroid rather than a scientifically determined cause of the enlargement, should still be the standard term used in the medical literature. However, the term can at least be narrowed down a little for purposes of this discussion. The goitre responding best to geographical analysis is simple endemic goitre, which is basically an enlargement of the thyroid gland arising because of lack of iodine in the diet. The gland in an attempt, as it were, to supply the body with the iodine it needs becomes over-stimulated, resulting in its enlargement to cause large swellings below the Adam's apple, often unsightly and sometimes seriously interfering with the functioning of such neighbouring structure as the trachea or windpipe, veins, nerves etc.

The thyroid is a two-lobed endocrine gland (or ductless gland, directing its product into the bloodstream) towards the front of the neck on either side of the Adam's apple. Several small parathyroid glands lie behind or embedded in the thyroid. The thyroid produces a hormone called thyroxine, a compound of iodine with an amino-acid (a weak nitrogenous organic acid closely linked with protein formation) which accelerates the release of energy from the combustion of glucose in the tissues. A fall in thyroxine levels in the blood stimulates the production of a Thyroid-stimulating Hormone (or TSH) in the pituitary gland (a ductless gland at the base of the brain, of complex functions mainly connected with growth and the maintenance of balance or feedback mechanisms in various bodily functions); the pituitary produces less TSH when thyroxine levels in the bloodstream are high. A second thyroid hormone, called calcitonin, operates a similar feedback mechanism when dealing with calcium levels in the blood—calcitonin lowers the calcium concentration, while the parathyroid gland raises it, the two by complementary controls maintaining an equilibrium in calcium content.

Simple endemic goitre, as noted earlier, arises basically from iodine deficiency (in the water people drink in a locality and in the food, and ultimately in the local soils if the food is mainly produced locally). This relation is the one mainly outlined below, but the thyroid gland's mechanism is relevant to our discussion, because it now seems clear that some simple endemic goitre is produced by goitrogens, or simply substances originating goitre; and it seems likely that some at least of these operate by inhibiting the use of dietary iodine in the thyroid to produce thyroxine by affecting some part of the complex mechanism described.[9]

Goitre has long been associated with particular areas, often inland areas, as witness Derbyshire neck, though the disease has in fact been common in a goitre belt from Derbyshire to Somerset and even to maritime Devon and Cornwall. Association with iodine has been directly or indirectly deduced, for the Chinese used seaweed, which contains iodine, as a medicine for it some 400 years ago.[10] More scientific studies enabled David Marine to declare in 1915: 'Simple goitre is the easiest of all known diseases to prevent . . . It may be excluded from the list of human diseases as soon as society determines to make the effort.' Marine was referring to his belief, soon proved in practice, that the great mass of the disease in heavily goitrous tracts could be cured or prevented by increasing the dietary intake of iodine—for instance, in salt. More recently it has been proved that, at least for bread-eating people dependent on bakeries, that the inclusion of iodine in the bread is a more effective way of combating endemic goitre.

The geography of simple endemic goitre was still justified as a major geographical study in a WHO monograph in 1960, and within a briefer paper in a recent volume of collected essays on environmental medicine.[11] Studies of contrasts in areal patterns of the disease have long been given additional point because of quite weighty circumstantial evidence that goitre may cause endemic cretinism—the more than random occurrence of births of babies wholly or substantially lacking in thyroid processes, or with gravely unbalanced ones, and stunted in growth, severely retarded mentally, and effectively deaf and dumb. Deaf-mutism and mental retardation without the major abnormality of thyroid development have both also been associated with goitre. However, the relations with cretinism, and particularly with other occurrences of deaf-mutism and mental retardation, are now doubted, and certainly not as linked with goitre in a very clear-cut way. Cretinism, it is now suggested, is more likely to be related to in-breeding than to goitre and iodine deficiency, and, like deaf-mutism and mental retardation, attributable to purely genetic causes.

Figure 64 is compiled from the WHO monograph of 1960. With its aid the world patterns of goitre will be reviewed.

The distribution of goitre is often attributed to dietary iodine deficiency, assumed to be related to iodine-deficient soils. Iodine deficiency in the soil is in turn attributed overwhelmingly to the Quaternary glaciation, which deprived very large parts of the world, in high latitudes or in high altitudes, of a fully mature, layered 'soil profile', which evolves over the course of some 5,000 to 20,000 years—faster in warm climates, slower in cool ones, and hardly at all in deserts. Differences in the mineral content of the immature soils are attributed to the parent rocks from which are derived the glacial rock-flour, boulder clay etc, or, presumably, water-borne outwash.

This attribution to glaciation is tenable for the USA, and one can only suppose a gap in the data as accounting for the sharp cessation at the international boundary at 49°N, with even more heavily glaciated Canada lying to the north. In Mexico and South America most of the goitrous areas can credibly be related to high mountain glaciation and some lowland tracts to glacial outwash. Similarly the pattern in Europe can reasonably be related to the Quaternary glaciation and its meltwaters and meltwater deposits. For this purpose, as for some others, we may include the Atlas mountains with the European pattern.

However, there are some puzzling anomalies: for instance, the inclusion of Devon and Cornwall in south-western England in the goitrous tract. These counties form a peninsula hardly exceeding 60 miles (100km) in breadth and in many places much less, and a markedly maritime environment in terms of winds and access to sea-food. Even recent work suggesting that the Quaternary glaciation extended further west and south than had been thought has not suggested a protracted glaciation of the whole of the peninsula. Peri-glacial activities may of course yield similar iodine deficiencies, but this does not seem to have been investigated.

The European pattern can be regarded as continued by the Urals and the Caucasus into Soviet Central Asia and by the Himalayan arc into eastern China and south-east Asia. Much of

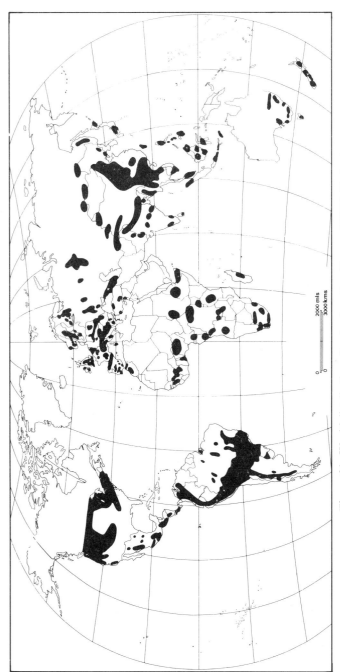

Figure 64. World distribution of endemic goitre. (Source: WHO. *Endemic goitre*, Monograph Series No 44, Geneva WKO, 1960.)

this can reasonably be attributed to glaciation, as it can in New Zealand—heavily goitrous in parts until iodized salt was made compulsory—and in south-eastern Australia. There some tracts are suggestive of the much older Carbo-Permian glaciation than the Quaternary one, and this may apply also to some of the goitrous tracts in the far south of Africa. Some of Australia's goitrous tracts, however, extend beyond the glaciated areas proper to areas that experienced only peri-glacial conditions, and, as suggested earlier, these may also induce iodine deficiency. The goitrous tract extends to the coast at Grafton, just south of the New South Wales/Queensland boundary, and it is difficult to believe that even alluvial deposits from rivers draining an iodine-deficient hinterland should extend and include deposits that must have been partly laid down under estuarine and maritime conditions and where iodine deficiency seems at first sight unlikely.

In Tasmania the goitrous tracts have at least at times extended beyond the area marked in Figure 64, which was certainly heavily glaciated, and while much of the island was glaciated during the Quaternary and the rest exposed to peri-glacial recent occurrences of goitre have pointed to goitrogens—that is, substances stimulating an attack of goitre. The disease was occurring in almost epidemic rather than endemic proportions. The goitrogen seemed to be the brassica (a plant of the cabbage family) fed to dairy cattle in the Tasmanian winter, which is sharp enough to cause seasonal shortage of pasture; in these circumstances the goitrogen was concentrated in the milk.

Looking at the world map as a whole, however, we notice that the glaciated and peri-glacial areas do not account for most of the goitrous areas of south and south-east Asia, and many of the old plateau surfaces of central Africa (excepting its highest mountains). Nor do they account for much lowland and plateau country in the Amazon basin, which may represent surveyed areas rather than actual patterns of goitrous tracts.

It seems essential to hypothesize a complementary cause to glaciation, but this is not easy, for the equatorial and tropical goitrous tracts include areas subject to a very wide range of climates, from constantly humid equatorial rain-forests through seasonally humid monsoon regions to semi-arid and arid tracts like Pakistan and south-west Africa. Perennial leaching seems a possible cause of iodine deficiency in rain-forest climates, and even seasonal leaching in areas of monsoon rainfall. But leaching out seems unlikely in semi-arid and arid areas, which, after all, include such areas of iodine concentration as the nitrate mining areas of northern Chile. Goitrogenic plants may be a cause.

It is tempting in a geographical survey, however, to look back at some pioneer work from India, still reviewed in modern literature surveys but not apparently taken very seriously. An important role was at one time attributed to calcium-rich water or soils, linking goitre not only with inland and often mountainous areas, as the text above does, but also with limestone tracts from Derbyshire to Kashmir. There is some classic detailed mapping and cartographic correlation of a major tract of the Indo-Gangetic plains in which goitre incidence is high and in which the variations appeared to be related to the calcium content of the alluvium derived from limestone-rich catchment areas.[12]

The pioneer nutritionist of India, Sir Robert MacCarrison, suspected that freedom from or liability to pollution of calcium-rich drinking water accounted for the difference between freedom from or common prevalence of goitre and, as well as experimenting on trout, he himself with other volunteers produced swellings of the thyroid gland in themselves after some weeks of drinking the polluted water (1906–8). This particular approach has seemingly been overtaken by events, with the very confident modern emphasis on iodine deficiency. However, even the present map (Figure 64) reveals puzzling anomalies, some of which have been noted earlier, and, as the many gaps are filled in, it may be possible and even necessary to review much of the earlier material, including some essentially geographical in approach, such as that by Stott *et al.*[13]

It may of course be necessary to repeat the survey work using more modern techniques, but if the differences recorded a generation ago were anything like accurate, the modern blanket explanations do not seem to cover all the facts. The more that is known about the real causes, the more effective are likely to be campaigns for prevention and cure of a distressing disease, which may still prove to be related to the appalling disabilities of preventable cretinism. Advanced countries have established control over goitre, as Marine was calling for in 1915, but in the Third World it remains uncontrolled over a much larger number of people than when he was issuing his pioneering challenge to preventive medicine.

Geographers and world food problems

A medical man turned geographer, the late Jacques M. May, compiled, partly with help from others, not just the ageing maps used in parts of this chapter but a massive series of bench-mark surveys of the state of nutrition and of knowledge about nutrition and malnutrition nearly all over the world.[14] There have been other, smaller contributions from geographers, including my own survey of kwashiorkor in the mid-1950s, in collaboration with Dr H. C. Trowell, used earlier in this chapter.

It is not a field where geographers' contributions to methodology or analysis have so far been very great, and yet the field seems to call for collaboration. Regional diets and dietary customs appear to invite geographical survey and analysis, and though Dr May repeatedly tried to interest geographer colleagues, there has been a marked timidity about following up his massive compilations. Is this because the field really calls for interdisciplinary team work? That can only arise, I think, in particular circumstances—perhaps by chance meeting of interested workers, who might make piecemeal advances but possibly invaluable progress in methodology; perhaps by major international effort, demanding substantial funds and diversion of effort from other research. The major attack might well be justified, but the case has not so far been made sufficiently strongly to attract support on the scale that would be needed.

Problems of geography and health in India often seem to stimulate effort, and Indian geographers have done a good deal of work on relations between land use and calories per head, mainly from Aligarh Muslim University. Some of this research, such as Dr Rais Akhtar's thesis referred to earlier, includes data on deficiency disease. Also from India comes the Tamil Nadu Nutrition Survey, the result of collaboration between the government of India and the US AID programme. This work is particularly challenging to geographers, none of whom served on the survey teams, because of its attempt to use a systems approach: food supply in Tamil Nadu was assumed to comprise a system with three sub-systems—food production, food processing and marketing, and food consumption. It used very large samples, especially in consumer surveys, and much more input from cultural anthropology than is usual in such studies; these characteristics enabled the team to be particularly clear about the vulnerable groups in the population—children on weaning, adolescent girls, pregnant women, lactating women are all especially liable to protein malnutrition—and about the extent to which their vulnerability persists even in comparatively prosperous strata of the population. It is hoped that wider 'action-research' programmes to follow will include geographical contributions, and that these will prove useful in remedial and preventive measures in India and elsewhere in the developing world.

CHAPTER SEVEN

Case Studies

Four case studies are intended to bring together the problems discussed separately in earlier chapters, and to do so in relation to specific areas, larger or smaller. There is a problem about case studies. Unless they are based on carefully designed sample surveys—unlikely in this field in the near future because of cost—they are not a suitable basis for generalization. On the other hand, the generalizations of earlier chapters are based for the most part on case studies, usually more specialist and less about general health than those in this chapter. To make a start one has to use the material to hand, and one often comes up against the problem of lack of comparability in the case-study material. Starting with two micro-regional or small area studies, we meet this problem at once, and later in the chapter it arises with our two nation-state or meso-regional case studies also; all four seem to me justified in the present context by their ecological insights. The micro-regional studies include one developing-world study and one from a developed country, though from a rural area.

The first study is of Wensleydale by the famous Dr William Pickles, the first President of the College (later Royal College) of General Practitioners, and arose from his work there before and soon after World War II; the second, of Kuwait about 1970, is by a medical man, Dr G. Ffrench, and a geographer, Dr A. G. Hill. The Kuwait study is largely concentrated on Kuwait city, in a state of very rapid change following the exploitation of petroleum; the other uses the fact that one can often see patterns in a small community that would be lost in a larger one—an approach already seen at work in Figure 8 (the flow patterns of infectious hepatitis in a small community in New South Wales) and Figure 45 (cancer in Horrabridge, Devon).

The two macro-regional studies are of Libya in the 1960s by Dr Kanter, a medical man; and of England and Wales from data mainly of the 1950s and early 1960s, from geographical studies by Professor G. M. Howe and others.

The Wensleydale of Dr Pickles

I recall a particularly lovely evening in early summer when I climbed alone to the top of one of our noble hills . . . And as I watched the evening train creeping up the valley with its pauses at our three stations, I had this strange thought, that there was hardly a man woman or child in all those villages of whom I did not know even the Christian name and with whom I was not on terms of friendship. My wife and I say we know nearly all the dogs and indeed many of the cats. Now, does not this intimate knowledge of his flock put the country doctor in a superior strategic position for the study of such a subject as epidemic disease? I could say much of my patients, the Yorkshire dalesfolk; of their shrewdness and ability; of their remarkable memories; of their startling intelligence, which tempts me to deplore that in some ways education blunts the edge of intelligence; of that seemingly impenetrable crust, which is only a crust, concealing great friendliness and goodness of heart. These are just the people to help a doctor in his investigations. Matters so delicate as heredity and consanguinity have to be approached with care, but on the whole I have found my patients co-operative and slow to take offence. Also, I cannot help knowing much about the details of their relatively simple existence. I have known the grandparents of many of my present-day patients and have been able to trace characteristics, medical and otherwise, through the generations to the present day. Today I know what markets the farmers frequent, the schools where their children attend, the young people's love affairs, the festivities that take place at intervals in every village of the dale, the visits to the large towns for shopping or the yearly expedition to the Pantomime and the summer trip to the seaside. On many of these expeditions, infectious disease has been introduced into our midst, and one is rarely in doubt

about the origin of any epidemic. A little help and encouragement turns the schoolmaster into an enthusiastic
epidemiologist, and I have been fortunate all these years in
having an ally, the headmaster of the grammar school, which
serves a large area and is often responsible for the spread of
epidemics.

There is, moreover, the stability and continuity of country
practice. Most of us show but little inclination to change our
habitat and retire with reluctance, knowing that our real life
is then over and fearing to experience that utter loneli-
ness which comes from a separation from our work and
from our friends. Not everyone has the temperament of a
Diocletian—content to throw away the purple and grow
cabbages and, as good students of Gibbon will remember,
even he lived to regret it.

If you are tempted to read some of Dr Pickles's work in the
original, his early and fascinating *Epidemiology in Country
Practice* is not too easy to find, but many major libraries have the
New England Journal of Medicine, which contains a splendid
brief account of his interests and methods, including the
retrospective passage quoted. He goes on to tabulate in order of
frequency the 4,855 cases of infectious diseases he has recorded
in just over 15 years, starting with influenza and diarrhoeas
including many Sonne dysenteries (caused by a bacillus), and 'at
the bottom, thank God, comes diphtheria'. His list includes
influenza, diarrhoea and vomiting, measles, febrile catarrh,
chickenpox, whooping cough, tonsillitis, mumps, German
measles, herpes zoster, hepatitis, scarlet fever, lobar pneumonia,
glandular fever, Bornholm disease, diphtheria, and erythema
nodosum. He pleads for medical students to be able to work in
general practice so that they can see this kind of mixture, as compared with the proportions of cases seen in hospital training
(Pickles helped to pioneer such an arrangement in the medical
school in Leeds).

It is worthy of note that, though doubtless the mortality of
Wensleydale was dominated by heart attacks and strokes,
cancers, and probably terminal pneumonia at times such as

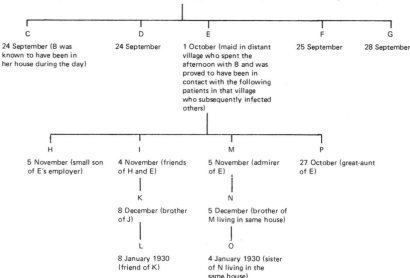

A (the first victim)

Not attended personally, but said to have had jaundice in July 1929. It is impossible to trace the infection in his case, but it is significant that he visited Askrigg, a hotbed of infection, in June.

B (A's sister)

Began with the disease on August 23 and while still obviously jaundiced, attended a village fete on 28 August. All those on the line below were also present and developed the disease on the given dates.

C — 24 September (B was known to have been in her house during the day)

D — 24 September

E — 1 October (maid in distant village who spent the afternoon with B and was proved to have been in contact with the following patients in that village who subsequently infected others)

F — 25 September

G — 28 September

H — 5 November (small son of E's employer)

I — 4 November (friends of H and E)

M — 5 November (admirer of E)

P — 27 October (great-aunt of E)

K — 8 December (brother of J)

N — 5 December (brother of M living in same house)

L — 8 January 1930 (friend of K)

O — 4 January 1930 (sister of N living in the same house)

Figure 65. Course of hepatitis among people in Wensleydale who attended a fête. (Source: Pickles, W. N. 'Epidemiology in country practice', reprinted by permission from *New England Journal of Medicine*, 239, 1948, Fig 1, p 420.)

influenza epidemic periods, Pickles's epidemiological, or here one may claim his ecological, work concerns infectious diseases and, especially so far as original research is concerned, their incubation periods. The examples of the hepatitis epidemic starting from a village fête has already been cited in Chapter 3. Figure 65 relates to the same outbreak and illustrates the method diagrammatically.

Dr Pickles goes on to a detailed account of his basically very simple methods, starting with a diary entry like 'March 10, 1947, Jonathan Metcalfe, aged ten, village of Aysgarth, measles', and thence to an entry on a chart like Figure 66, arranged by 'natural' groupings of villages for a quarter; names and brief clinical notes were recorded opposite, and the sheets of graphs filed in books,

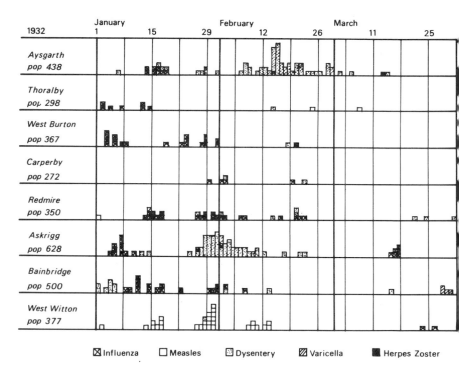

Figure 66. Example of Pickles's epidemiological records in Wensleydale. (Source: as Figure 65, Pickles, Fig 3, p 422.)

adding up to a remarkable but simple data bank concerning the flow of infections through Wensleydale. (We learn from E. M. Pemberton's biography of Dr Pickles that much of the recording was done by Mrs Pickles.)

The scientific contribution was largely on incubation periods of infections, some being established by Dr Pickles, and some confirmed from laboratory work by reference to his 'natural laboratory'; always, in this context, it was the 'short and only possible exposure' that he was seeking: the man who found the surgery closed, crossed to the inn for a drink meanwhile, then reported and was found to have measles, which he had given to a fellow drinker; the boy with measles who was kept isolated at home but infected an aunt by means of a peculiar long window connecting his bedroom and a living room with the family meal table beside its lower end; the rather sick little bridesmaid who went down with mumps after the wedding, the bride succumbing 15 days later.

Dr Pickles then discussed the major epidemic of influenza, the strain of making, say, fifty epidemic calls a day in a rural area, including many isolated farms, while still caring for other patients (some of them 'malades imaginaires'); he suggests that by the 1937 epidemic there were noticeable effects of improved transport and the closing of village schools in favour of larger central ones, which he believed added to the spread of the infection: 'It gives us visits to isolated farms that otherwise might have escaped and many walks in the midst of strenuous days over sodden fields, not at all acceptable.' Figure 67 shows part of an epidemic in 1935: a schoolmistress returning from the Christmas break with her parents in Scarborough, and feeling unwell, nevertheless dutifully persisted in teaching on the first day of term—and was responsible for seventy-eight cases in her pupils and their families, though also for a low rate of infection in that community in the 1937 epidemic, owing to immunity from two years before. This was one sequence Dr Pickles discussed with the great Australian virologist Sir Macfarlane Burnet, leading to work on the charts proving considerable community immunity for 4 years but fading completely in 7. Then there is the case of the schoolmistress who spent the autumn half-term holiday in Manchester in 1943, and infected several pupils on her return to Wensleydale while there

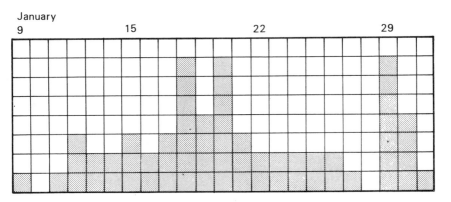

January
9   15   22   29

Figure 67. Influenza in Wensleydale, January 1935. (Source: as Figure 65, Pickles, Fig 4, p 423.)

was still no sign of a countrywide epidemic, which was to rise to 1,300 cases a week by the end of the year—an example of the 'pre-epidemic seeding' of Chapter 3.

The relation between chickenpox and shingles or herpes zoster was under discussion and Figure 68 shows a sequence starting with a young mother with supra-orbital herpes on 27 April, then her baby daughter on 31 May developing chickenpox, which spread through school and on to a sister village; the herpes case on 15 July lived in a very isolated farm indeed, and the only possible source of infection was a visit from a small girl who only afterwards developed the chickenpox rash, so must then have been infectious. So on to the series (not illustrated here), starting with almost simultaneous illness from shingles of a young married woman and a farmer 4 miles off, explained by an innocent link a fortnight earlier—a farm sale in the farmer's village, and an invitation to the woman to come home for tea with her friend, the

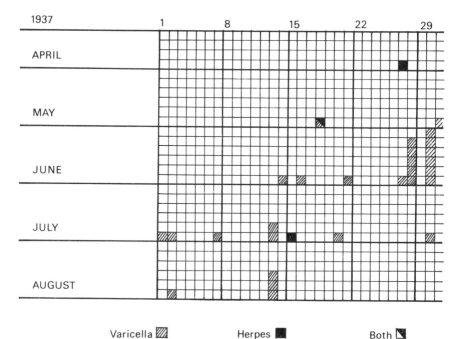

Figure 68. Chickenpox and shingles in Wensleydale, 1937. (Source: as Figure 65, Pickles, Fig 5, p 424.)

farmer's wife. The farmer, undeterred by shingles, attended the tea and sports for King George VI's Coronation and infected nine people with chickenpox and one with shingles, and one of them infected his grandfather, who had shingles. Even in summary the flavour of Dr Pickles's down-to-earth epidemiology probably comes through, but read him in the original if you can!

The last 30 years have seen many changes affecting the kind of community represented by Wensleydale. Rural populations making their living from the land or serving those who do so have further declined with mechanization. The way of life of all has been affected by transport changes—the advance of the cheap motor bus, the decline of the railways, and then the decline of the bus as private cars increased to cover almost all except the old and the poor in rural communities. Shopping facilities in small towns have gone down, with the ease and speed of car travel to major centres for shopping—for range of choice of 'comparison goods' and cheapness of many items of daily shopping needs in the supermarkets. There is the decline in the village schools, noted by Dr Pickles as making for more rapid spread of infections in the larger schools to which country children are taken by school bus. There is the national health service, increasing the effective demand for medical treatment, and within it on the whole the decline of the cottage hospital and the greater importance of the more centralized regional hospitals.

The movements of people are more rapid from day to day, and from year to year, too, for the villager who has never been outside his native place is now a rarity, and an ageing one. So patterns of movement of infection are more complex, and more difficult to trace, though it is still worth doing so where fresh light can be thrown on a disease of importance to public health, like infectious hepatitis, for example. Population migration may make it more difficult to study the environmental relations of comparatively slowly advancing diseases like cancer. But it is probably true that studies like those of Dr Pickles can still be worth while, and are more likely to be so if they can be linked with ecological models similar to, but preferably better than, those discussed earlier in this book. Greater mobility of population is an impetus towards the 'cohort' type of analysis already in use for particular purposes. This consists of following through the subsequent health history of a particular group of people, such as those born in a particular town in a particular year. There could well be applications in medical geography both for those who stay on in the same place and for those who travel. Are there differences within the town, and differences between the immobile and the mobile people?

Kuwait

A book on Kuwait written jointly by a medical man, G. Ffrench, and a geographer, A. G. Hill, allows me to include an unusually widely based study in this chapter.[1] While it covers the 40,000sq km of Kuwait's territory, it is naturally concentrated on the city of Kuwait, which in 1965 contained almost 300,000 of the country's 470,000 people. At the same date non-Kuwaitis accounted for almost 250,000 people—increasing to almost 450,000 in 1968—and for a large part of the increase from the 1904 population of some 48,000 (about 13,000 Badu or Bedouins, and 35,000 settled cultivators and townsmen).

Kuwait is a small Arab State, lying near the head of the Persian Gulf, on its south side, with its northern border only some 60km south of Basra, the Shatt-al-Arab and the joint delta of the Euphrates and Tigris. Its geologically young rocks, from the Eocene to Recent, include the oil-bearing strata and structures that account for the world importance of this small country, and which have also supported the recent rapid population increase and immigration, together with the very rapid urbanization, modernization and urban redevelopment programmes. Moreover oil revenues have financed a quite remarkable scale of health provision, including excellent sewage disposal in fully sewered areas—a model for sanitary engineers from other Middle East countries.

While the country, Kuwait city and the oil towns make this case study a special one, there are lessons for poorer developing countries; indeed, as Ffrench and Hill claim, Kuwait is 'an epidemiological sounding board for the Middle East'. Modern development is superimposed upon an age-old picture of contrast between wandering and often warlike Badu (Bedouin) herdsmen, the settled cultivators of fields and date gardens, and the city—one of the smaller trading centres in a strategic head-of-gulf situation in a civilization where cities are immemorial, and where we need not expect the urban models of Chicago to apply. We have to look for a health picture in transition from Arab medicine of traditional scholarship on the one hand, and Badu hygienic customs on the other, both dominated by such hygienic provisions of the Old Testament and the Koran as the forbidding of pork as a food and the low esteem in which the dog is held.

Rapid urbanization and the flow of immigrants from different cultures are occurring in one of the hottest urban environments in the world, with relative humidities up to but fortunately not often exceeding 50 per cent on the stickiest days. Temperatures fall almost to freezing point on many winter nights, and there are only short spring and summer interludes when outdoor activities can be described as pleasant. Rainfall over 20 years of reliable records has never exceeded 20cm (about 8in), so water supplies have always been a vital topic, from oasis waters to modern bore-wells to tap fossil water (naturally of variable quality with different aquifer rocks) and now desalination plant. In the modern city streets, where redevelopment has all but swept away the traditional thick-walled brick or mud-walled courtyard town house, the noise of air conditioners is the most constant of city sounds. But the influx to the city is such that poor immigrants to an oil-wealthy capital do not escape what Ffrench and Hill call pseudo-urbanization—the shanty towns on the edge of the city so common from Indonesia to Brazil.

Urban ecology in Kuwait City
A statistical analysis carried out on the social ecology of Kuwait City was based on 'factor analysis' of thirty-eight variables, available by census enumeration districts. Some of these might be expected to vary in sympathy (to 'co-vary'), so that further analysis of a small number of 'key variables' would in fact carry into the research the effects of the several groups of co-variates. The thirty-eight variables analysed are listed in Figure 69, and those were reduced to eight groups of co-variates, and finally to Factors 1, 2 and 3, as mapped in Figures 70–2. Such quanti-

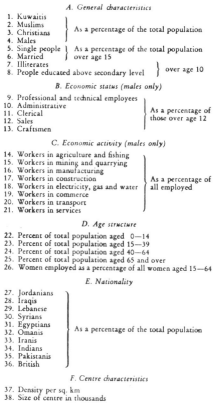

A. General characteristics

1. Kuwaitis ⎫
2. Muslims ⎬ As a percentage of the total population
3. Christians ⎪
4. Males ⎭
5. Single people ⎱ As a percentage of the total population
6. Married ⎰ over age 15
7. Illiterates ⎱ over age 10
8. People educated above secondary level ⎰

B. Economic status (males only)

9. Professional and technical employees ⎫
10. Administrative ⎪
11. Clerical ⎬ As a percentage of those over age 12
12. Sales ⎪
13. Craftsmen ⎭

C. Economic activity (males only)

14. Workers in agriculture and fishing ⎫
15. Workers in mining and quarrying ⎪
16. Workers in manufacturing ⎪
17. Workers in construction ⎬ As a percentage of all employed
18. Workers in electricity, gas and water ⎪
19. Workers in commerce ⎪
20. Workers in transport ⎪
21. Workers in services ⎭

D. Age structure

22. Percent of total population aged 0—14
23. Percent of total population aged 15—39
24. Percent of total population aged 40—64
25. Percent of total population aged 65 and over
26. Women employed as a percentage of all women aged 15—64

E. Nationality

27. Jordanians ⎫
28. Iraqis ⎪
29. Lebanese ⎪
30. Syrians ⎪
31. Egyptians ⎬ As a percentage of the total population
32. Omanis ⎪
33. Iranis ⎪
34. Indians ⎪
35. Pakistanis ⎪
36. British ⎭

F. Centre characteristics

37. Density per sq. km
38. Size of centre in thousands

Figure 69. Kuwait: table of thirty-eight socio-economic variables. (Source: Ffrench, G. E. and Hill, A. G. *Geomedical monograph series, Regional studies in geographical medicine*, Vol 4, *Kuwait: urban and medical ecology*, New York, Heidelberg, Berlin, Springer–Verlag, 1971, Table 28, p 43.)

tatively founded analyses give a firm basis of reference to health indicators such as infant mortality in relation to particular population groups.

Factor 1, or Kuwait citizen factor. Of the total variability, 38·7 per cent is explained by the distinctive characteristics of the Kuwait population. A very young population, they have a high proportion of married people and a very high rate of natural increase, encouraged by the government; they work largely in service industries and are nearly all Muslims. They are seldom craftsmen or construction workers. This group dominates in the Kuwaiti suburbs of Kuwait city (9–15 in Figure 70), and in

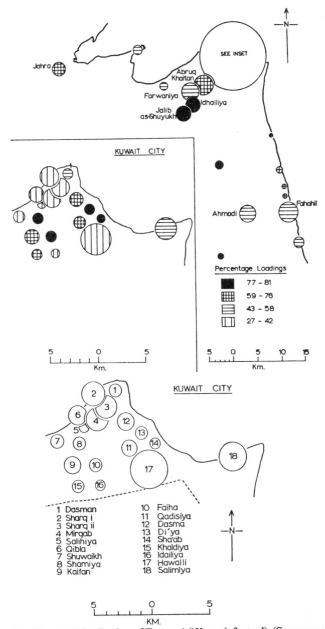

Figure 70. Kuwait: Distribution of Factor 1 ('Kuwait factor'). (Source: as Figure 69, Ffrench and Hill, Fig 18, p 45.) Inset: Urban centres, 1965, and suburbs within Kuwait. (Source: as Figure 69, Ffrench and Hill, Fig 12, p 42.)

villages in the south and east of the country. They are conspicuously lacking in the Old City and in the oil settlement of Ahmadi.

Factor 2 or high-status non-Kuwaiti factor. These better educated immigrants are also very largely Muslims who are employed in craft or commercial, but not manual, occupations; they are predominantly male and married (many having left their wives in their country of origin). This group is concentrated in parts of the Old City (Figure 71) and avoids the Kuwaiti suburbs and the low-status immigrant areas. Their distinctive characteristics account for 25·2 per cent of the total differences in the thirty-eight variables of Figure 69.

Factor 3 or low-status non-Kuwaiti factor. These groups

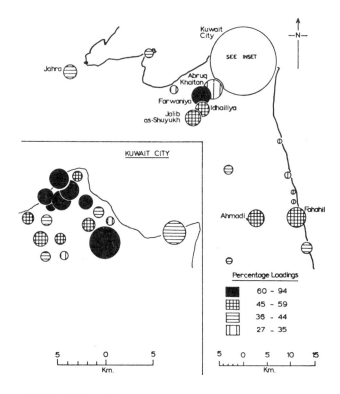

Figure 71. Distribution of Factor 2 ('High-status non-Kuwaiti factor'). (Source: as Figure 69, Ffrench and Hill, Fig 19, p 45.)

account for 28·1 per cent of the total variation. Poorly educated immigrants, largely Irani and Iraqi and frequently illiterate, they fall mostly into the young and active age groups engaged in construction or craft activities, and do not live in large centres. They generally occupy temporary housing or hutments wherever construction work is afoot, and in industrial areas (Figure 72).

The end product gives an indication of distinctive socio-economic groups within the population which may or may not form an identifiable spatial pattern of 'social areas' within the city. While much of the spatial pattern has emerged in relation to these three factors, it is worth noting that the Old City contains a good many high-status non-Kuwaitis in some areas, including British, Americans, Pakistanis and Indians (almost 27,000 of the Old City non-Kuwaiti population of 70,000 in 1965). Then there are substantial areas dominated by married non-Kuwaitis of medium status, including Jordanians. While most areas have few low-status non-Kuwaitis, major individual projects like the building of the Hilton Hotel increase this Factor 3 component.

Ffrench and Hill point out that the importance of areas of different ethnic groups is by no means unusual in Asian cities, including of course the important shanty-town areas. The concentration of Kuwaitis in Kuwaiti suburbs could be matched from elsewhere, but the radical redevelopment of the central city and the great importance of recent immigrants from neighbouring countries are unusual, and seem to me to impart an unusual character to both the Old City and the shanty town areas.

Health and rapid urbanization in an oil-rich society
The stresses of rapid transition are dramatically presented by the example of Badu burial and defecation practices, the former in a pit very near the family tent, the latter anywhere in the sand around the tent. The faeces rapidly lose offensiveness and pathogenicity in the dessicating and antiseptic sunshine, and arouse dormant desert grass with unwonted shade and moisture. While the transition to towns is easy for the wealthy Badu, rapidly becoming educated in urban ways, these practices clearly are subject to drastic change even among poorer Badu spending at least some period in the shanty towns, as do other immigrants,

who may come from less contrasted environments than do the Badu.

Adult Badu may be thought of as survivors of high infant and child mortality, exposed to comparatively few infections beyond those to which they have acquired immunity in childhood, and therefore leading healthy adult lives on into old age. In towns they may well be exposed to unaccustomed dangers, such as intestinal infections spread from cesspits and open sewers in shanty towns, in contrast with the rapid neutralization of faeces in the desert. Or again urbanizing Badu may fall rapid prey to obesity and other troubles of sedentary urban man. Much of the ecological interest of this research lies in this theme of distinctive patterns of urban adjustment and urban stress, not just of Badu, but of other immigrants with lesser traumas—from around the Persian Gulf, or, the authors suggest, from a comparably harsh environment in

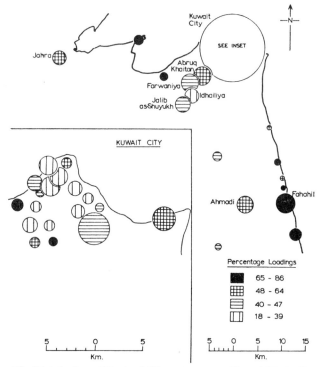

Figure 72. Distribution of Factor 3 ('Low-status non-Kuwaiti factor'). (Source: as Figure 69, Ffrench and Hill, Fig 20, p 45.)

Texas, or from very different environments in the Levant or in South Asia.

Vectored infectious diseases
Really arid climates inhibit fly-breeding generally, though flies are quick to take advantage of favourable seasons or times of day, or locally friendly environments, even on a very small scale. So the traditional Badu way of life was comparatively free from many of the vectored infections of underdeveloped countries. The old city gave a different environment and plague, for instance, has a long history here. The old close-packed streets, like many from the Levant to China, made good rat warrens, and ancient trade routes connected Kuwait with the market cities of the Indo-Gangetic plains, their periodic epizootic and epidemic peaks replenished in turn from the enzootic 'silent zone' of the disease among the marmots of Central Asia. Plague, though a human disease of great historical significance is ultimately a zoonosis. Plague appears to have a recurrent long-term cycle of rise and fall. A period of falling incidence seems to have coincided with the widespread use of DDT and other residual insecticides during World War II and in post-war India for instance. India probably has no more plague cases annually at present than arise from the 'silent zone' in the desert mammals of south-western USA. Other rat-borne infections have not been serious in Kuwait, and Ffrench and Hill suggest that rat tunnels in house walls support a comparatively light rat infestation as compared with cities like Basra, with sewage pipes and tunnels harbouring large rodent populations.

Schistosomiasis or bilharzia, one of the great scourges of the developing world, depends on the fluke/water-snail/man cycle. It is common in the Basra delta and rare in an arid tract like Kuwait, and the full cycle is likely to remain so unless Kuwait's water shortage were to be solved by digging a canal from the Shatt-al-Arab—a solution naturally opposed on health grounds. There is, however, an odd human problem of oil-based prosperity: the male dominance in immigrants such as the Factor 3 group is linked with an inflow of brides, many from bilharzia areas in the delta, and the sexual activity following the arrival of a long-awaited bride causes a flare-up of the uro-genital symptoms, and of course quite serious stresses and delay in the arrival of eagerly expected children.

Returning to vectored zoonoses, leishmaniasis occurs in Kuwait in two forms, cutaneous and visceral leishmaniasis, both carried by sandflies. Cutaneous leishmaniasis is a disease of desert rodents carried by *Phlebotomus sergenti*; man blunders into the zoonosis when man–sandfly contact is close, near rodent burrows in the desert, which also harbour the vector, but this seems seldom to occur in Kuwait, though there is a small incidence reported among students, higher in winter and low in the hot dry weather unfavourable to arthropod life in the open. Visceral leishmaniasis or kala-azar, if untreated, is a serious recurrent fever and often kills. Urbanization, increasing sophistication in way of life, and the loosening of Islamic taboos on the dog, the primary host of the pathogen, are increasing the keeping of dogs as pets and also the risk of kala-azar. The local vector is *P. papatasii*, which seeks a combination of shade and damp such as is found in broken-down buildings and the like. The 'clear-felling' type of urban development that has transformed much of the Old City has led to the dumping of bulldozed rubble around the edge of the city; these dumps both breed the sandfly and are attractive to dogs, so spreading the enzootic cycle to people within flight range of the sandflies.

Non-vectored infections

To follow through dog-keeping into this fresh category of disease, the change from dogs guarding camps and hunting (the Saluki is a local breed) to dogs as pets has brought other risks. Where dogs, livestock and people live together, even under conditions apparently much more hygienic than in Kuwait, there is a risk of hydatid disease, in which man becomes caught up with the life cycle of the dog tapeworm *Echinococcus granulosa*, often with serious effects. Eggs excreted with the dog faeces may be ingested by livestock, or find their way into man's intestinal tract through poor personal or food hygiene. A common way in which the cycle is perpetuated is by dogs feeding on parasitized meat, often mutton; it can be broken by cooking scraps fed to dogs, but this has proved difficult even under Australian conditions, for instance. New infections in Kuwait are showing a high rate of increase and, though numbers are comparatively small, the effects can take a long period to show, and the impact of this change in old customs is to be taken seriously. Rabies is not found, but does occur in surrounding countries, so again the change in custom carries a serious risk.

Another zoonosis, toxoplasmosis, is a parasitism of the tissues of many species of mammals, including man, birds and some reptiles, by the sporozite stage of the protozoan *Toxoplasma gondii* (cf the malaria cycle), the only known complete host being the cat—though it seems unlikely to be the only one in fact—but the mode of transmission to man being unknown. Normally the presence of the protozoan in human tissues seems harmless, but in a small proportion of pregnancies it causes stillbirths or congenital deformities, including blindness. This infection was investigated in Kuwait partly to probe the idea that transmission might be by insects or other arthropods—it had so far been mainly associated with humid areas—and partly in relation to traditional and potential contacts between man, stock and domestic animals. While pathogenicity was rare, and prevalence rates in surveyed population not suggestive of a large public-health problem, it was comparable with other areas of moderate endemic and enzootic conditions in more humid areas, like much of Queensland, with a much wider range of arthropods that might be vectors. Expansion of stock-rearing would raise the question of toxoplasmosis control in animals.

In respect of the universal infectious diseases Kuwait remains generally fortunate, though Ffrench and Hill think that the comparative freedom from non-virus infections may be fragile in a time of change in the society. In water-scarce Kuwait water-borne disease is not common, though it includes light incidence of typhoid. Non-venereal syphilis, recorded from comparable environments in surrounding countries, is not important, nor the spirochaetal infection known as relapsing fever. Amoebiasis as an active disease is not common. Amoebic ulceration of the intestinal tract is a not uncommon disease, and a proportion of cases seem to occur when *Entamoeba hystolica* acts pathogenetically; this selective pathogenic impact is suspected to be connected somehow with modern urban-industrial stresses, and it is puzzling that in the west ulcers seem to attack particularly the colon, with more cases in women, whereas in Arabia, including Kuwait, there are more cases among men, and it is the rectum more often than the colon that is ulcerated. The introduction into previously austere modes of life of tinned food and a more luxurious diet has been suspected as a factor, as has the much greater use of drugs.

On the other hand, the dust and overcrowding in some communities have brought severe virus epidemics: measles is a serious scourge of children, causing many deaths in poor areas; influenza was severe during the pandemic of 1957 analysed for Britain in Chapter 3; and smallpox has caused a sharp epidemic as recently as 1967, though world control of this most severe virus disease appears imminent at the time of writing. Skin disease in school populations showed a wide variety of infections, with a maximum in winter and a minimum in the hot dry summer, but they appear to be within normal limits for a country still with a wide range of environmental hygiene. The proportion of venereal diseases, notably gonorrhoea and syphilis, was over 1 per cent of the population studied, and was regarded as disquieting, especially since syphilis in students seemed to be concentrated among Kuwaitis, possibly in association with alcoholism and drug addiction. In non-student groups non-Kuwaitis predominated and venereal diseases were less, presumably because of the large male predominance in the large immigrant population.

Non-infectious causes of ill-health
Genetic disease included blood abnormalities like the sickle-cell trait, which is evidence of the former extension of malaria, even though it has not been widespread in Kuwait in recent decades. There is some evidence that consanguineous marriages were related to higher proportions of congenital defects, and rates are high by world standards, with little difference between Kuwaiti and other groups.

Accidents include a growing toll from the roads, particularly among young men, and there is a link with alcohol consumption, despite prohibition, in relation to illicit stills and to driving back to

Kuwait after journeys across the border to Iraq to drink there. Industrial accidents, including burns due to explosions in tankers and risks of pollution and major disaster, are closely monitored by oil company occupational medicine. Heat exhaustion and other effects of heat are of course well known but not common, thanks to very careful study and precautions. In well-to-do populations air-conditioning plays its vital part, but it can break down, sometimes through industrial action, and a sharp rise in the incidence of heat exhaustion in new immigrants in shanty towns and in tanker crews some years ago has now been controlled by education campaigns and the wide availability of remedial measures.

Psychiatric breakdowns are comparable in numbers with western experience, or with that in Egypt, a major Arab country from which pyschiatric skill is drawn; this is worth mentioning because even Egyptian psychiatrists record difficulties in making contact with their patients in Kuwait, and also marked differences in types of breakdown. Incidence seems to be higher among Kuwaitis than among other groups. There is some suggestion that the apparently high incidence of homosexuality attributed to the seclusion of women in purdah in Islam is related to the high prevalence of neurosis, and this is commonly accompanied by paranoia in townsmen but not in Badu. Schizophrenia is thought to be hebephrenic (characterized by giggling or silly or bizarre behaviour) more frequently than in comparable populations in Egypt. Urban populations are thought to have a particularly high incidence of delusions, and it is thought that the stresses of urbanization play a part—and possibly the stresses of industrialization also, more specifically those connected with very rapid growth in responsibility accompanying rapid 'Arabianization' in the petroleum industry.

Lessons from Kuwait
Kuwait data point to the presence of psychological difficulties in 74 per cent of patients (lack of security, family and financial difficulties, fear of cancer), to infections in 44 per cent (amoebic, bacillary and schistosomal), to food sensitivity in 6 per cent, to purgatives in 6, and to no obvious factors in 10. Clearly there is

often overlap, eg between infections and anxiety. Gastro-enteritis
of infants and children is a serious cause of illness and death, as in
any population in the developing world where there are wide
disparities in community hygiene, piped water and sewerage,
prosperity, housing and education; and the wide if unequal diffusion of wealth in Kuwait does not exempt her from this scourge.

A comparison between two hospital catchments is partly
vitiated by non-comparability in the two populations: one is the
government hospital in Kuwait, where the population is regarded
as unselected (though even there poorer communities may suffer
in silence rather than expose themselves to the alien environment
of a hospital), and the other the oil company hospital at Ahmadi,
which deals with a population necessarily selected by occupation,
income, and cultural orientation, and biased by the tighter
environmental control possible in a company town. Nevertheless,
the former's 1,000 odd patients included about 500 Kuwaitis and
67 deaths, whereas the latter's 60 patients included only 19
Kuwaitis (32 per cent compared with 53 per cent), and only one
death. Ffrench and Hill urge the encouragement of early
attendance at clinics even at the risk of overloading them, on the
ground that preventive paediatrics can still be very effective under
such pressures.

Looking back over their study, Ffrench and Hill consider their
'epidemiological listening post' in relation to infectious diseases.
The relatively fortunate position of Kuwait among developing
countries comes out in many ways. One example is that while
blindness is around the world level of about 1 in 20 of the population, comparatively few blind people are in the younger age
groups now, and cases resulting from infections are of decreasing
significance as control of trachoma, measles and smallpox is
established and residual cases from these causes pass into older
age groups. However, the incidence of glaucoma is now an
increasing problem.

This change in the epidemiological picture is of the kind that
justifies the claims by Ffrench and Hill that Kuwait represents an
epidemiological sounding board for the Middle East. From the
viewpoint of this book on medical geography, I hope that this
account has given some fresh material on the ecological side for

the reader's world view of the constant change and mobility in the filling of ecological niches, and also some instances of the impact of movement of people, and of urban development, on the more geographical side.

Ffrench and Hill note broader implications. Dualism, for instance, is often thought of as a characteristic of colonialism, but it survives into thoroughly nationalist phases in that there are still two worlds within 'Arabianized' Kuwait—people who are living in the European style and at European standards of education, hygiene etc, mixed with the 'pseudo-urbanized' and rural poor. Ffrench and Hill plead that much education is misdirected, neglectful of the sciences which, carefully applied, can assist Kuwait to prosper and to enjoy prosperity rather than be harmed by it; but the presence of malnutrition even amid wealth is an example of the type of problem caused by dualism and failures of education and communication to cross cultural barriers. They note that loyalty to very widespread leading families may squeeze smaller and less powerful ones, and that the pockets of malnutrition in the midst of plenty are a warning; if such vicissitudes as epidemics of infectious disease can lead to malnutrition, then for many the margins between health and disease are too narrow for a prosperous and civilized country. Ffrench and Hill admire, as who cannot, the splendid hospital and laboratories, and elaborate occupational and preventive health service, and think they may well be appropriate in wealthy Kuwait, with an average annual income around 1970 of £1,000 per head, no income tax, petrol at 5p or so per gallon, and electricity and water almost free or at minimal charges. But they doubt its wide applicability to developing countries, even to developing Arab countries as a whole, except for the wealthiest, which means the other oil producers.

For this book are there any additional points? The ecological insights are fascinating, throwing light on many less fortunate areas of the Third World. To broaden from the ecological to the spatial patterns is not really possible from a single case study; but it is at least safe to say that this Kuwait study makes one very cautious about the *deus ex machina* type of health provision as compared with some approaches that are a little slower and, as it were, more rooted in the local soil. As in many parts of the book, my own view is that it points to the need for advances in health and health services to be part of all-round social and economic development programmes, preferably locally activated though without deliberate blindness to lessons from elsewhere in the world, developed or developing.

Libya

One of the sister volumes to the Kuwait study deals with Libya, and is written by a medical man using a great deal of the method traditional in regional geography.[2] This study, like that on Kuwait, still covers a largely desert and Muslim state in which petroleum has recently become of prime importance to its 1·6 million population and to the world market. The area is very different, however, from Kuwait, for Libya is a land of almost 1·8 million sq km, extending from the north-eastern part of the Sahara in Fezzan to the mediterranean terrain of Tripolitania and the largely limestone country east of Benghazi in Cyrenaica, the two areas with substantial mediterranean cultivation being separated by a long stretch where desert and date-palm oases reach the sea.

If the coastal belt is on the semi-arid fringe of mediterranean climate and agriculture, impressive ruined classical cities and irrigation works—the latter partly reactivated—testify to the importance of the area in Greek and Roman times. A long period of Turkish control gave way to an Italian colonial phase from 1912 to World War II, when the coastal belt in particular was much fought over. Substantial agricultural and irrigation development or redevelopment, with many Italian colonists, began during the Italian phase. Some tens of thousands of Italians remained on in independent post-war Libya, at first under the puritanical Islamic rule of kings drawn from the Senussi nomadic herder and warrior tribes of Fezzan, and latterly under the similarly puritanical Muslim dictatorship of Colonel Gaddafi.

Apart from the larger area, the coming of petroleum exploitation of the Tertiary rock structures south of Benghazi has led to a more complex interaction between nomad and oasis cultivator, Italian colonist, old and new towns and cities, and puritanical Islamic culture. The weight of Dr Kanter's analysis lies much

more towards the rural population than in the study of Kuwait,
and the best way to give the flavour of his treatment is to quote
from his chapter called 'Region and Disease: Geomedical
Conclusions',[3] referring to his interesting regional map
(Figure 73):

> The Libyan area has been divided into 26 regions,
> differentiated according to the nature of their surface and of
> their climate and thus also of their hydrological conditions
> and their plant cover. Except for small sections of the pop-
> ulation, the inhabitants of the country are of one uniform
> culture and live in the landscape component parts most
> suited to their needs, some of them as farmers or

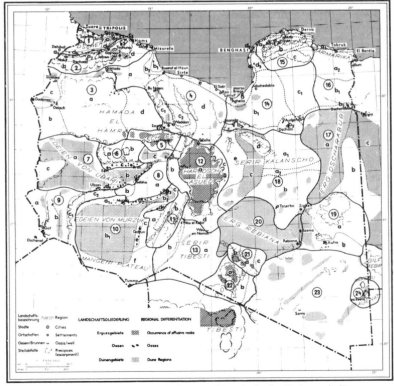

Figure 73. Libya: regions and landscapes (*Landschaftsgliederung*). (Source:
Kanter, H. *Libya: a geomedical monograph*, Heidelberg, Academy of Sciences
and Berlin, Springer–Verlag, 1967, Map No 3, folding.)

townspeople in consolidated settlements, which means close to one another, others scattered over the country as semi-nomads, often linked with a permanent settlement but in the main wandering around in order to make use of the less favourable regions. Today only a small section of the population may be considered as pure nomads. A number of regions are scarcely utilizable and are therefore devoid of people, so that in comparison with the size of the country the population lives only in a few regions and again chiefly in smaller sub-regions of these. The enormous scale of the area, the long distances between individual settlements and the still difficult communications all play a part in determining the condition of health of the population. It is a country that does not encourage the rapid spread of epidemics. On the other hand, general conditions of health are impaired by endemic infectious diseases, above all by '*nestling epidemic diseases*' (Jusatz) which are at home in the region independent of man and transmitted to man by insects, water and/or foodstuffs. The question which arises here is in how far a dependence of these diseases, as for example in the cases of malaria, the leishmaniases, dengue and others, can be attributed to the regions in Libya.

This regional relation can be demonstrated with some of the vector-borne infections, including zoonoses, and then to some extent by man-to-man infections.

Vector-borne infections, including zoonoses
This dependence, Kanter reports, is clear in respect of malaria. The adjustment of the malaria cycle of Chapter 4 to conditions in Libya is discussed. Breeding of the vector *Anopheles* occurs most importantly after the winter cool period, when it takes advantage of the later of the depression rains, which feed bodies of water, sunlit or shaded, running or still, according to the breeding preferences of particular species. *A. maculipennis* prefers sunny still water at 22–29°C, and other species brackish water in coastal lagoons or swampy flats between sand-dunes, puddles in hollows in sand deltas at wadi mouths, pools behind strand-banks, and

water in the leaf-axils of palm fronds. Irrigation ditches and furrows and drainage areas may contain water for long enough to promote anopheline breeding. A period of about 4 weeks of favourable conditions in spring leads to biting by females in late February, and the malaria cycle is established if there are 3 weeks or so with temperatures over about 16°C, lasting through summer. *Anopheles* avoids hot dry conditions by crepuscular activity, and attains an autumn peak in November before declining to a winter trough of activity, when it hibernates in cracks in rocks and walls, palm-front fences, *maquis* vegetation and the like.

In Figure 73 regions 1a, 2f, 4e, 14a, 14d and 16a are broadly malarious, with exceptions, as in the Zuara area near the western border, where coastal lagoons appear to be too saline for anopheline breeding, some having linking channels to the Mediterranean. Long shunned as malarious, except for temporary tented nomadic settlements and small towns, this belt is the site of three new oil-exporting ports that will require careful planning and surveillance to avoid malaria. There are risks of malaria spreading inland—for instance, into such low plateau areas as region 4d—if water is ponded back from the coastal region. On the other hand, the Italian colonial period showed that control could be effective even before modern insecticides were available, as round Benghazi ($14d_1$ and d_2). Even quite low coastal hills, as in regions $1d_1$ and $15a_1$, have higher rainfall, with risks of malaria along spring-lines and seepages, while the low plateaux have high run-off or rapid seeping into limestones. The true deserts of the south and south-east (regions 18–24) and even southern Tripolitania (region 3) have a climate hostile to *Anopheles* and only small oases, round which irrigation gradually salinizes the soils so that bodies of water are not attractive to breeding females; however, new artesian wells present some risk of extending malaria (eg Gadomes in Region 3c). In the Fezzan (major region 6) climate and hydrology are in places favourable to the vector, with numerous fresh-water wells and irrigation channels, and long wadis with lines of oases, so that traffic is brisk and the reservoir of human infections is renewed. Elsewhere, as in region $10a_3$, for instance, oases are poorer in water and more ıne from another, so that risks are lower.

The mosquito-borne virus disease dengue is carried by the culicine mosquito *Aëdes aegypti,* which is also the domestic vector of yellow fever (see Figure 3). In Libya this is a mosquito of land under 600m preferring hot summers but humid mild winters. It has become very closely adapted to man, though it also bites other animals, and breeds in every sort of stagnant water—rain gutters, open wells, irrigation ditches, and discarded cans —allowing the larvae 10–14 days for development in rainy spells. The eggs are able to lie dormant when need be for several months, ready to hatch at the first shower. Mild winters followed by hot summers and mass invasion of houses by this day-biting vector may lead to epidemics anywhere in the coastal regions, and while the influenza-like illness used to be comparatively mild, it is recently showing signs of increasing in severity in some parts of the world.

Schistosomiasis or bilharzia, already encountered in Kuwait, is an important disease, mainly in parts of Fezzan (major region 6), where the molluscs find favourable conditions in open wells, deltas, irrigation ditches and artesian wells. Areas like Wadi Edri (region 7d$_1$) are, however, too saline for the mollusc, or water is simply too scarce; and similarly in southern Tripolitania the cycle exists in some oases like Dersh (region 3b) but Gadames is free (3c), apparently because its large artesian well is walled in and kept clean. The Tripoli region (1a) has long been regarded as at risk unless swamps are drained etc, because of the chance of infection by caravans or pilgrims, and later by shanty-town immigrants from the Fezzan. Similarly, in Cyrenaica, coastal areas with perennial water like Derna (region 15a$_1$) are at risk from infected travellers, and also major water sources in the plateau inland, visited by nomads who seem to be a strong source of infection. Farther south, however, oases like Marada (region 4b$_2$), Jaghbub (17), Jalo (14b$_3$), and Kufra (19b) seem to be too saline for the snail or too isolated to support the disease cycle.

Typhus, a louse-borne rickettsial infection, is a case of vectored human disease that Kanter classes as a shifting epidemic—as opposed to a nestling epidemic (see below in relation to relapsing fever)—shifting among desert nomads, especially in winter, when warmer clothes are worn and kept on at night as well as by day, and shifting among the susceptibles—mainly children, with adults mostly immune (see Figure 74). Lice may also carry relapsing fever, caused by a spirochaetal *Borrelia*, though it also seems that this disease of desert rodents, foxes etc may be carried to nomads in camp by ticks of the genus *Ornithodurus* living in clefts and cracks of caves and houses and in sandy soil. The disease sometimes travels in camel bales in caravans to the coastal cities, as in 1912, 1933 and 1942–44. Since this is primarily a disease of desert mammals, an enzootic, it can be viewed as a nestling epidemic, in contrast to a shifting epidemic like typhus.

Plague has been a significant disease; it also can be a nestling epidemic related to an enzootic, as it is in Central Asia. Kanter

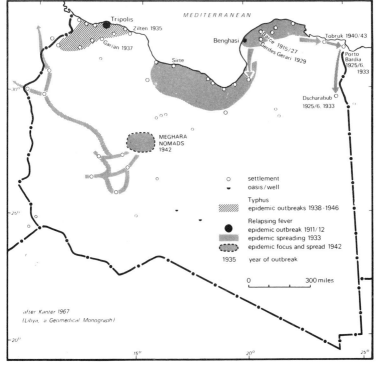

Figure 74. Libya: typhus and relapsing fever, 1911–46. (Source: as Figure 73 Kanter; and Learmonth, A. T. A. 'Medicine in medical geography', in McGlashan, N. D. [ed]. *Medical geography: techniques and field studies*, Methuen/University Paperbacks, 1972, Fig 2–5, p 32.)

says it is mainly a shifting epidemic here, but it occupies an intermediate position. It has repeatedly been imported to the seaports,
for instance, or by the caravan routes across the desert, but has
been spread via the nomads to the desert rodents. Thus the disease
seems to have been imported to Benghazi (region 14) in 1917, and
was significant as an urban epidemic until 1922, but lingered on as
a rural shifting epidemic related to the peculiar secondary
enzootic until 1940. Tripolitania had a similar though apparently
quite separate epidemic history at about the same period. The
desert climate and even most of its microclimates are basically
hostile to the rodent fleas that transmit the bacteria, but since they
could travel in caravans, they can just as easily travel long
distances by modern lorry traffic if another major plague cycle
should occur.

Continuing with the vector-borne zoonoses, cutaneous and
visceral leishmaniasis, already noted in relation to Kuwait, are
important in Libya. *Phlebotomus* of some sixty species breed in
walls of ditches and canals, wild rodent burrows, and humid
decaying organic matter and the like. The protozoal parasite is
found in dogs, cats and rodents, and man is brought in where
man–sandfly contact is close—when a man rests near rodent
burrows, for instance. The true desert is sufficiently hostile to the
sandfly for it probably not to be important south of about 30°N, ie
in the southern three-quarters of Libya. Though in a different
category on present knowledge, in that man is the only known
reservoir of infection, we should note that the sandfly is also a
vector of sandfly or pappataci fever, a virus disease with
symptoms like dengue or a mild influenza.

Zoonoses not dependent on vectors but spread more directly,
mainly in milk of cattle and coats in nomads' herds, include the
bacterial brucellosis and the rickettsial Q-fever or Malta fever.
Kanter records probable import of infections from Malta, Sicily
or Egypt, and yet the acquisition of some immunity by the
nomads.

Non-vectored infections
Moving to diseases transmitted by man-to-man contact, or sometimes by mechanical transport by house flies etc, Kanter finds

some association with region and culture. The interaction of trachoma and bacterial eye infection noted in Chapter 4 gives a good example. Under conditions of poor hygiene, desert oases have widespread trachoma infection, and flies concentrated in oases and in freely watered and well dunged fields (to avoid the arid sterility of the hot summer in the desert) also spread bacterial eye infection over wide areas. There is a peak of incidence in the autumn date harvest, and keratitis associated with malnutrition, especially vitamin A deficiency, adds to the many crippling eye disabilities.

Again deliberate or accidental spreading of human manure on damp irrigated fields, and defecating in fields, in warm temperatures for most of the year, make for intensive development of helminthic infections often debilitating. Amoebic and bacillary dysenteries are widespread, and there is a substantial typhoid problem where there are local or imported carriers.

One must add to Kanter's picture of non-vectored infections the universal diseases like influenza, measles and pneumonia, the skin diseases, the malnutritions in underprivileged groups and so on, and remember the movement and change from desert nomad and from oasis and Mediterranean cultivator to an oil-exporting country.

From the point of view of this book this particular case study brings to life the ecological approach to infectious diseases of Chapters 2–4, and in an environment of wide vistas across desert to mediterranean landscapes, in a country always of mobility, and now of complex interaction, including ex-colonial and new petroleum interests. The traditional geographical approach of the regional concept is used. The reader may judge the extent to which this approach has been followed through into the medical geography, and how far it has been linked with the medical ecology.

Health and health services in England and Wales

For the last case study I have chosen to discuss regional disparities in health and health service in England and Wales. As in previous case studies, its availability at a particular time dictates the use of more or less dated material in order to set out a method or approach to the data. In discussing England and Wales I shall draw on work by G. M. Howe,[4] and some by B. E. Coates and E. M. Rawstron,[5] from a 1972 Open University 'second level' course called 'Decision making in Britain'.[6] Some of the maps concern material originally gathered by the registrar-general round the mid-1950s, though processed and published in map form some years later. I think I can say that all the authors quoted in this way would join with me in regretting that there is no continuously available and up-to-date 'weather chart' (Rawstron's phrase) of health and health services (and of related socio-economic patterns). Computer mapping and cheap format publication could be done at modest cost once a programme was evolved, and the reader may judge for himself from this case study and preferably from the original works cited whether or not work along these lines would justify the necessary effort and cost.

The following treatment of some of Professor Howe's maps is adapted from teaching rather than research writing by the present author. By including this I am able to make some points about possible geographical approaches that cannot otherwise be made. At a simple level we shall go beyond the visual inspection of maps so often used earlier in the book, to testing a hypothesis, in this case a descriptive rather than a causal-analytic one, using an elementary statistical test. Despite the out-of-date material and the simplicity of the approaches, the reader may catch a glimpse of the potential that lies in regular analysis of health and socio-economic data, costly as maintaining Rawstron's 'weather chart' would be. Professor Howe's maps, already simplified in this book as Figures 43–6 and 50–1, use standardized mortality ratios—standardized to allow for the different expectation of death from all causes, or for a particular disease of young people or old age, or of one sex, according to the age and sex structure of the population in different areas. (Figure 1 also comes from his atlas, but differs because infant mortality is measured in relation to the numbers of live births.)

This standardization procedure is explained in the discussion of Howe's maps of cancer in Chapter 5. Many of the maps used in this book refer to Howe's 1954–58 data, published in 1963, rather than to his later information, because his 1970 atlas, covering the years 1959–63, uses maps on a demographic base, similar to that employed by Hunter and Young in Figures 11 or 12. While the demographic base map has many advantages, it is not easy to collate the distribution pattern with that in other maps with which the map reader might want to make comparisons. Where Professor Howe has made available a conventional map using 1959–63 data, this map has been used. In pulling together into some regional generalization certain findings placed before us all by Howe in his two atlases, I drew a rather crude and arbitrary division between macro-regions (or major regional divisions) within England and Wales, simply calling them North and West, on the one hand, the South and East, on the other (Figure 75). One may work at the maps, using the relatively low-level hypothesis *that the North and East are disadvantaged in health and in health services compared with the South and East*. The statistical test used, chi-squared or χ^2, can be followed in the captions to the relevant figures. It is applied here by comparing expected and actual incidence of fifty random map references falling on the two regions. We should stress that this simple area-sampling technique carries its own bias, it emphasizing area and not, say population, but one has to start somewhere.

A first group of maps may be thought of as giving some indications of general health, supporting the hypothesis that the North and West of England and Wales are disadvantaged. These are Figure 1, infant mortality; Figure 75, deaths, all causes, males (the map for females shows less strong contrasts within the two regions, but is still weighted towards the North and West); Figure 76, accidents, females (the map for males is broadly similar but with a wide spread of moderately high rates in much of the South and East); and Figure 77, suicides, males (the map for females is broadly similar but with fewer of the high rates in the North and West, and more in the Greater London area and in a few other parts of the South and East, such as parts of East Anglia). While there are variations in the tabulated scores on the simple plotting exercise and χ^2 test, there is a broad pattern of heavy rates in the North and West. The 1970 atlas maps for 1959–63 broadly corroborate these findings, though the demographic base maps enable one to allow for smaller populations (eg in North Wales),

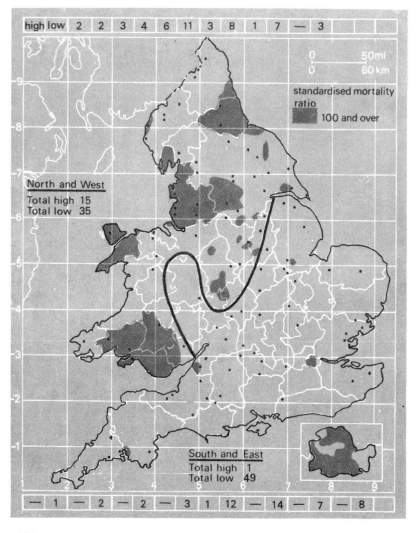

Figure 75. England and Wales: mortality from all causes, males, 1959–63.
Taking this as one index of general health conditions, and accepting my
arbitrary division of the area into a North and West of England and Wales, and
a South and East region, there is some indication on visual inspection of
adverse conditions in the North and West. (Source: Howe, G. M. *National
atlas of disease mortality*, RGS/Nelson, 1970; and Open University. *D203
Decision-making in Britain*, Block 5, *Health*, Bletchley, Open University
Press, 1972, Fig 3, p 33.)

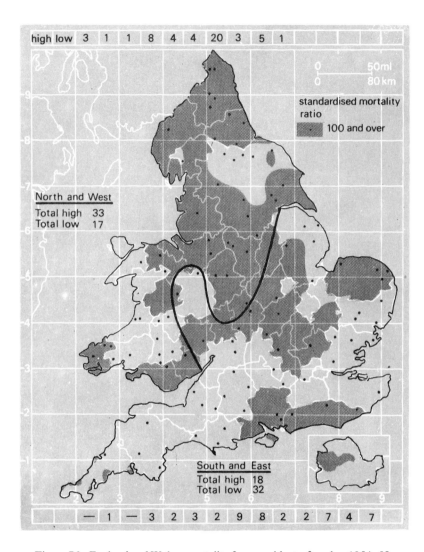

high low 3 1 1 8 4 4 20 3 5 1

standardised mortality
ratio

▓ 100 and over

North and West
Total high 33
Total low   17

South and East
Total high 18
Total low   32

— 1 — 3 2 3 2 9 8 2 2 7 4 7

Figure 76. England and Wales: mortality from accidents, females, 1954–58.
Readers may be surprised to see that there is some bias towards higher
incidence in the North and West, though unlike some maps with this bias
northern and western Wales are comparatively light and South Wales is high;
and there are some surprisingly high rates in the South and East, in the East
Midlands and East Anglia, and in several contiguous counties on the south
coast. On testing with χ^2, the bias towards higher ratios in the North and West
appears significant at a probability of 95 per cent. (Source: as Figure 75,
Howe, and Open University, Fig 7, p 39.)

198

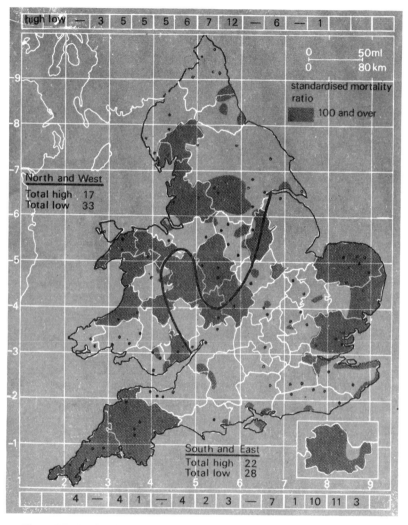

Figure 77. England and Wales: suicides, males, 1954–58. There is some bias towards higher rates in the North and West of England and Wales, using an arbitrary division, but another westerly area not included in this has high rates, namely Cornwall and Devon, and there are high rates in rural East Anglia as well as in parts of London. Using the χ^2 test, the bias towards higher rates in the North and West is not significant. (Source: as Figure 75, Howe, and Open University, Fig 8, p 40.)

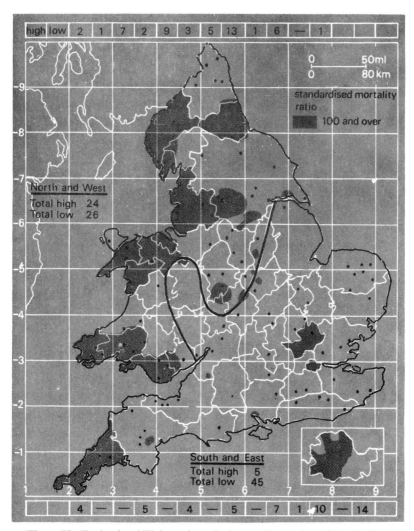

Figure 78. England and Wales: tuberculosis mortality, males, 1954–58. The bias towards higher ratios in the North and West resembles Figure 55 of bronchitis mortality rather than Figure 46 of lung cancer deaths. The χ^2 test confirms this, on the evidence, at 99·9 per cent probability. (Source: as Figure 75, Howe, and Open University, Fig 11, p 45.)

and note which symbols are regarded as statistically significant in their difference from the national expectation. There are also some maps where changes are recorded, though whether at random or as part of a tendency over time is not clear on present analyses: for example, suicide for males appear to have increased in the Greater London area in particular, and the later map for females resembles the 1954–58 map.

There are differences in data mapped. Road accidents, for instance, are given in 1959–63 as against all accidents in 1954–58, where the very numerous accidents in the home will appear.

A second group of diseases is related to the respiratory organs: Figure 50 for bronchitis, males (the map for females is similar, but lower in the Lake District, Snowdonia and Cornwall); and Figure 78 for pulmonary tuberculosis, males (the map for females is similar, and both 1959–63 maps are compatible in pattern). The map of lung cancers (Figure 43) for males has already been discussed in Chapter 5. The maps of bronchitis and tuberculosis support the hypothesis that the North and West are disadvantaged but, while there are high rates of lung cancer in the North and West, another factor, such as cigarette smoking, seems to be at work, as noted earlier; and there are many high rates, particularly in urban areas in the South and East. The later maps and the maps for females broadly support these findings, though one is continually reminded that within the South and East there are disadvantaged areas, such as parts of London, particularly the East End.

A third group of maps lends some support to the general hypothesis, including perhaps more surprising diseases. Cancer of the stomach in females is mapped in Figure 44 and the map for males, not reproduced here, is broadly similar, but with fewer very high ratios in Tyneside and the Midlands, and rather more in central and north Wales. The maps for 1959–63 are less strongly weighted towards the North and West. Cancer of the uterus (Figure 45) also lends some support to the hypothesis, and it seems that generally poorer housing, hygiene and genital hygiene may play a part.

According to the Howe atlas maps of arteriosclerotic disease, including coronary disasters, and of vascular disease of the central nervous system, including 'strokes', there are plenty of high risk areas in the South and East yet some weighting towards the North and West. If there is anything in the hypothesis that soft water is related to vascular disease, there may be some support here, but this is a topic on which findings are contradictory, and much more work would be needed before stressing it. Howe, in more detailed research of 1970 following up his national atlas work, has pointed out puzzling discrepancies in heart disease within Glasgow, yet the whole area draws its soft water from Loch Katrine. Could this be related to more old lead plumbing in poorer parts of the city, soft water having greater power to dissolve lead?

In addition to lung cancer, just discussed, others of Howe's maps seem not to support the hypothesis. Diabetes for females (not reproduced here) is only weakly concentrated, if at all, in the North and West, while the map for males (not reproduced) is broadly similar but with more high ratios in the South and East and fewer in the North and West. Cancer of the breast (Figure 46) does not share the bias towards the North and West of cancer of the uterus. Is there more breast feeding in the North and West, or was there at the time of these data? Other maps not supporting the hypothesis (not reproduced) include pneumonia, and gastric and duodenal ulcers, for both 1954–58 and 1959–63. The reader may wish to refer to the 1970 atlas for himself (it includes the 1954–58 maps and the 1959–63 ones), for the utility of my simple descriptive hypothesis, the small number of my random map references, and the suitability of the χ^2 test for this purpose may be questioned. But there is enough indication that the North and West are disadvantaged in health indices—or were at the time the data were recorded—to justify further serious work and serious thought, to put it at its lowest level.

I have often been asked why medical geographers have seldom followed up such spatial analyses by studies designed to solve particular problems. While I think there is a case for specialized studies on a narrow front—perhaps on the relation of bronchitis to indoor rather than outdoor pollution, for example—there may be a kind of echo of the repetitive theme that emerged from Third

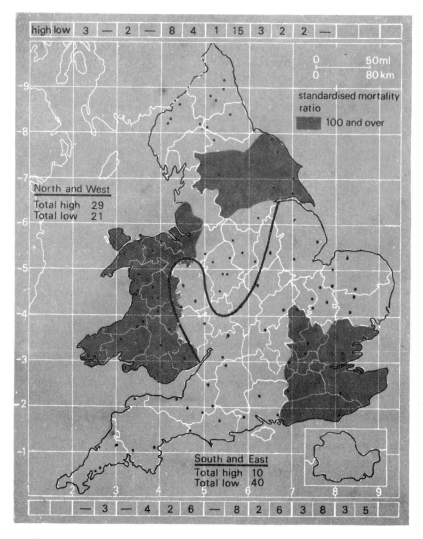

Figure 79. England and Wales: hospital beds used per million people, 1963. Visual inspection suggests some bias towards higher hospital usage in the North and West of England and Wales, the χ^2 test giving a probability of 99 per cent, so that such bias in sample points does not arise through chance. (Source: Coates, B. E. and Rawstron, E. M. *Regional variations in Britain: studies in social and economic geography*, Batsford, 1971; and Open University. *D203 Decision making in Britain*, Block 5, *Health*, Bletchley, Open University Press, 1972, Fig 17, p 52.)

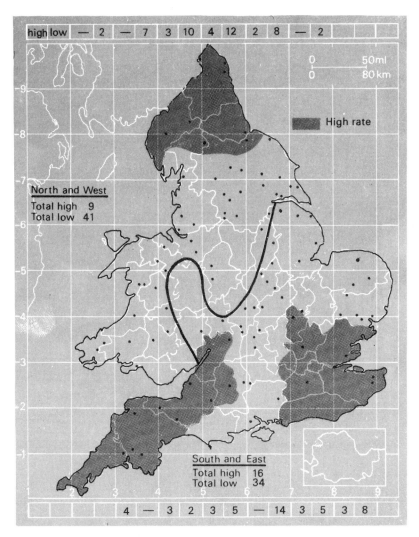

Figure 80. Hospital costs per patient by Regional Hospital Boards. There is some indication of generally high rates in the North and West of England and Wales, but this is offset by a group of contiguous areas of high rates around and east of London, so that our random map references and the χ^2 test here yield very inconclusive results. (Source: as Figure 79, Coates and Rawstron, and Open University, Fig 17, p 53.)

204

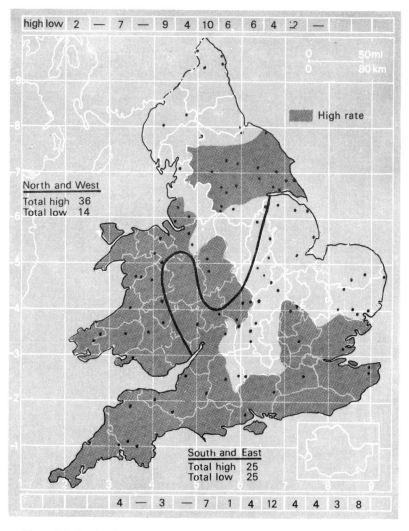

high low	2	—	7	—	9	4	10	6	6	4	2	—

High rate

North and West

Total high 36
Total low 14

South and East
Total high 25
Total low 25

4	—	3	—	7	1	4	12	4	4	3	8

Figure 81. England and Wales: male mental-hospital resident patients by Regional Hospital Boards. My North and West regions of England and Wales show if anything lower rates than the South and East region, but the distinction is not clear-cut on visual inspection or on inspection of the high and low sample points, while χ^2 does not show significant differences. (Source: as Figure 79, Coates and Rawstron, and Open University, Fig 18a, p 54.)

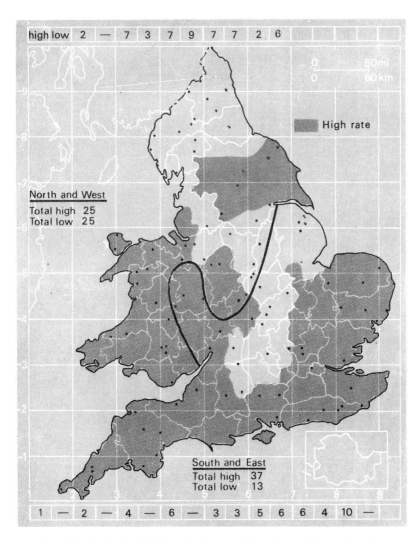

Figure 82. England and Wales: female mental-hospital resident patients by Regional Hospital Boards. Here my South and East regions show distinctly higher rates than the North and West of England and Wales, while the χ^2 test here shows a 10 per cent chance of this bias arising by chance. (This is regarded as not significant.) (Source: as Figure 79, Coates and Rawstron, and Open University, Fig 18b, p 55.)

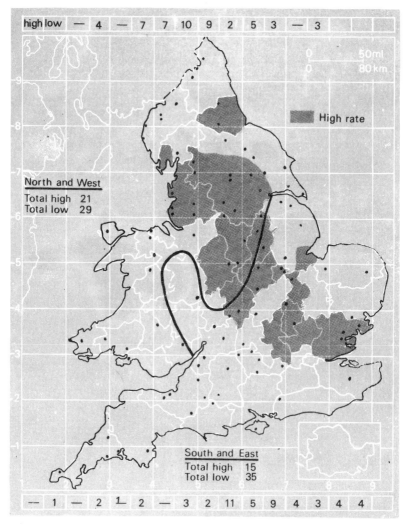

Figure 83. Average list size of general practices. Note that low list sizes may be regarded as favourable. High rates are characteristic of neither the North and West of England and Wales, nor of the South and East region, but rather of a belt or ridge across industrial England, and the sample points and χ^2 test confirm that the slightly higher number of points could fall on the North and West region purely by chance. (Source: as Figure 79, Coates and Rawstron, and Open University, Fig 19, p 57.)

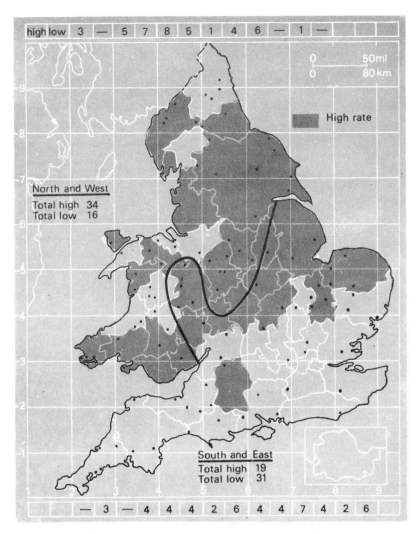

Figure 84. General dental service by counties. Again lower rates are more favourable, and visual inspection suggests slightly more favourable conditions of dental care in a sort of south coast region rather than in the South and East region, while the North and West region does have some areas of comparatively low and favourable rates. The sample points suggest slightly more favourable conditions in the South and East, while χ^2 suggests weak significance (at 95 per cent level). (Source: as Figure 79, Coates and Rawstron, and Open University, Fig 21, p 57.)

World studies, which stressed the need for development of the physical and socio-economic environment, with up-grading of the economy, housing etc in disadvantaged areas, rather than piece-meal investigations and answers.

Turning to the health services, we find that the available maps are much less satisfactory for the exercise than were Howe's mortality ratio maps. They are all based on a challenging book by Coates and Rawstron, and the various administrative regions for

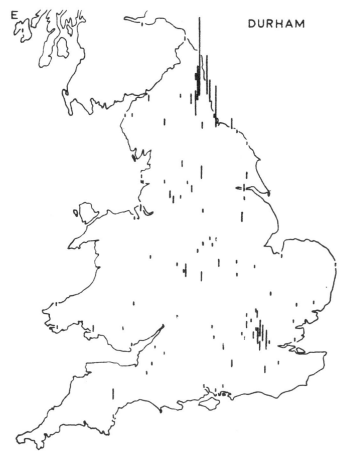

Figure 85. Dispersal of dentists from general qualification: Durham graduates. (Source: as Figure 79, Coates and Rawstron, and Open University, Fig 23a, p 61.)

different health-service purposes at the time were in general too broad. However, in Figures 79–84 using the random dot exercise and χ^2 test as before, we see a much less clear-cut picture than in the group of disease maps that do quite strongly support the hypothesis. An exception is the map of dental provision, Figure 84, with a markedly favoured area stretching right across southern England, though our arbitrary regional division includes in the South and East region a group of disadvantaged counties in the East Midlands and the northern part of East Anglia.

It must be stressed that these studies were carried out before the recent changes in the organization of the National Health Service, which turned away from 'historical budgeting', in which low past spending was apt to be linked with low future spending, towards budgeting in relation to population and need. They are not anything like so indicative of a kind of 'underdeveloped' North and West, but they do show a very patchy and irrational kind of variation. Shannon and Dever[7] review the National Health Service in Britain in terms of 'muddling through', and despite benefits most British people feel they have received from the NHS over the past generation, these maps make one wonder if that judgement is right after all.

In demonstrating a geographical approach, which might be deepened in operational and practical terms, Chapter 7 has taken us to the theme of medical care geography. That is further developed in the concluding chapter of the book.

CHAPTER EIGHT

Conclusion: Towards a Geography of Medical Care

The case study of England and Wales in Chapter 7 extends into the geography of health care, and the interested reader will find that there is a considerable literature concerning the United Kingdom or parts of it. In the USSR, again, ecological and health-care aspects of work appear to be closely integrated, in new settlements in Siberia and Soviet Central Asia, for instance, but more generally health-care aspects are left to the administrative hierarchy—discussed later, using the findings of ecological medical geographers but without intimate cross-disciplinary links.

However, a treatment of this topic in this concluding chapter of this book is justified largely because of a fresh stream of work and thought from the USA during the last decade or so, though, as noted later, some crucial work was done in Sweden around 1960. The American work is part of the impulse towards greater 'relevance' that has motivated many younger workers in particular in recent years. While a proportion of geographers have always found a commitment in the application of geography to practical problems in the community, there is now a fresh sense of commitment to a geography much more radically devoted to changing society, to something much more akin to what is sometimes called social engineering. The demand for relevance in this sense has brought some valuable books and papers, of which two in particular are used in this section.[1]

Enthusiasm for this approach has turned some geographers,

possibly a little impatient with the older ecological medical geography, towards a more 'relevant' medical care geography, as they see it. While understandable, two considerations arise from this reaction: first, that good ecological medical geography may assist in the prevention of disease, as suggested in my introduction, and second, that the greater the understanding of the ecology and space relations of the disease or disease complex concerned, the better is likely to be the forecasting, the logistics, the planning for medical care viewed spatially. Of course the operation is apt to become unwieldy if one cannot begin to plan the location of a new health centre without understanding, for instance, the cell biology of each range of cancers—all presenting complex problems, and the knowledge about them increasing, changing, in a state of flux. Still there can be moderation in all things.

There seems every reason to suppose that the two streams are complementary, and this is apparent in the work of Pyle and of Shannon and Dever. Moreover, both streams can be refreshed and reactivated by flows from the whole stream of geographical research. At the risk of repetition, it seems worth stressing that this is in one sense the vital reason why professional geographers, interested in mainstream geography, should study medical geography.

Health-care geography in the USA

Shannon and Dever wrote their book[2] specifically as a response to a time of agonizing reappraisal of health-care delivery in the USA when, on some indicators, the country was falling behind in the control of infant mortality, diseases of old age and various others, despite rising costs of health provision. I shall summarize their argument.

Medico-geographical detective work has a long history: witness the now often cited map of cholera in the Soho district of London, published in 1855 by Dr John Snow, in which the cases were shown to be clustered round a polluted well and pump, and ceased when the pump handle was put out of action. The more modern type of ecological medical geography, seeking links with spatial analysis and with various models (such as spatial diffusion models), are too seldom linked with geographical analysis of medical care patterns. Examining the varied patterns of provision of medical care—the complex patterns of private medicine and insurance provision and payment in the US, in contrast to the national health services of the USSR, the UK and China—we can see these as varying considerably with history and politics, with national genius and mores, with stage of economic development and perceptions of ill-health. The health-insurance principle is more compatible with private-enterprise economies; and the provision of health services as part of the whole governmental provision of social services is more compatible with socialist ideals and command economies.

The trend is probably towards government intervention and planning, even in private-enterprise or mixed-economy countries, simply because of increasing costs. As soon as planning is brought in, the question of rational spatial organization arises. As for other market provision, a theoretical model can be deduced of health provision on an isotropic plain, that is, a plain uniform in all respects, including population distribution and availability of

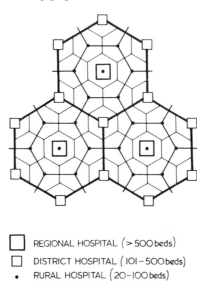

☐ REGIONAL HOSPITAL (> 500 beds)
☐ DISTRICT HOSPITAL (101 – 500 beds)
• RURAL HOSPITAL (20–100 beds)

Figure 86. An 'ideal' health delivery model (ie assuming uniform distribution of population and complete freedom of movement across the area in all directions). (Source: Shannon, G. W. and Dever, G. A. *Health care delivery: spatial perspectives*, New York, McGraw–Hill, 1974, Fig 2.1, p 12.)

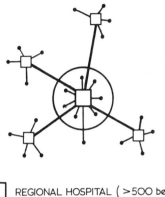

REGIONAL HOSPITAL (>500 beds)

DISTRICT HOSPITAL (101-500 beds)

• RURAL HOSPITAL (20-100 beds)

Figure 87. A 'realistic' health delivery model (ie removing assumptions of Figure 86 to allow for different sizes of settlements, channelling of movements across the area, and an area repelling human settlement. (Source: as Figure 86, Shannon and Dever, Fig 2.2, p 13.)

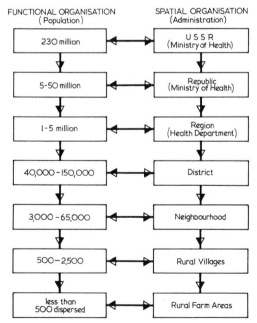

Figure 88. Spatial functional organization of health care in the USSR. (Source: as Figure 86, Shannon and Dever, Fig 2.3, p 15.)

transport in all directions (Figure 86). Geographical readers will realize the relation with Christaller's model of central place theory.[3] In contrast to the theoretical is a 'realistic model' more adjusted to the heterogeneity of the real world (Figure 87).

The hierarchical arrangements of the health services of the USSR, as shown in Figure 88, are aimed at complete integration with national planning. The advantages of complete coverage have to be weighed against the disadvantages, notably lack of choice and the reliance of the lowest rungs of the hierarchy on the *feldshers* (field workers), able to care for about 1,000 people. The *feldshers* can diagnose and treat patients, though they are not

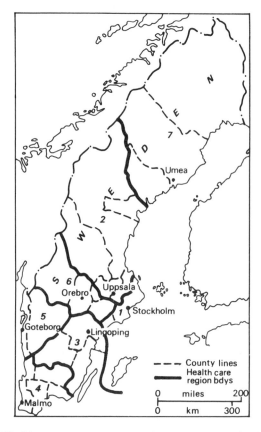

Figure 89. Health care regions of Sweden. (Source: as Figure 86, Shannon and Dever, Fig 2.4, p 19.)

medically qualified, and can call on the services of a qualified doctor at the neighbourhood level, the third bottom rung of the ladder. (In recent international discussion about medical geography workers from the USSR appear to find it difficult to sympathize with the concern for 'relevance' of American medical care geographers. For them the hierarchy of medical care will cope with all needs.)

The long history of health provision in Sweden includes a complete reorganization in 1960, when geographical analyses were used.[4] There is a four-level hierarchy of provision of higher level facilities at regional centres, familiar enough in principle but distinguished by consciously geographical spatial analysis (Figure 89). Stockholm gives an example of larger scale analysis of a small area of high population (Figure 90).

The National Health Service in England—presumably meaning the UK—is rather patronizingly regarded by Shannon and Dever as 'muddling through' to attain a more defensible spatial organization. (This judgement has, in fact, been overtaken by new areal arrangements, following the reforms of the health services in 1974.)

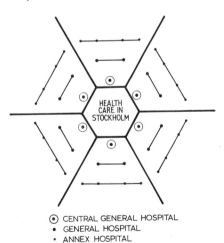

CENTRAL GENERAL HOSPITAL
GENERAL HOSPITAL
ANNEX HOSPITAL

Figure 90. Intra-urban health delivery model in Stockholm. This is presumably 'ideal' like Figure 86 but capable of approximation in the real world, ie in Stockholm, more along the lines of Figure 87. (Source: as Figure 86, Shannon and Dever, Fig 2.6, p 22.)

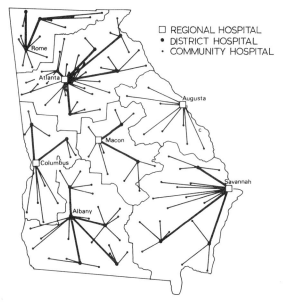

Figure 91. Regional health delivery model, Georgia, USA, 1970. (Source: as Figure 86, Shannon and Dever, Fig 2.10, p 31.)

The position in the USA is not so much a 'non-system' as a pluralistic, or partial, system with several identifiable sub-systems. There are the prepaid group practices, and medical care foundations (non-spatial organizations rather like 'friendly societies' in which health provision is obtainable to enrolled members in return for subscriptions, without altering the fee-for-service basis of medical practice). There is the more recent and rather more broadly conceived Health Maintenance Organization, which may include prepaid group practice or a medical care foundation but attempts broader planning of health care delivery and power for the enrolling population. Then there is the idea promoted by the American Hospital Association that each major geographic area should have at least one Health Care Corporation, aiming to combine local allegiance and planning with the advantages of central allocation or organization of territories etc, after the fashion worked out spatially for Georgia in Figure 91 (this is regarded as sufficiently centralized to attract opposition from the American Medical Association).

A review of the very broad distribution pattern of health resources in the US—physicians, hospitals, laboratory facilities etc—is comparable with the latter part of the case study of England and Wales in Chapter 7, allowing for differences in the size of country and political arrangements etc. For various reasons it is not easy to compile really detailed maps of standardized mortality ratios, but, by viewing maps by states and some earlier pioneer mapping,[5] one can see that higher rates tend to cluster in the southern states, as do, perhaps unsurprisingly, infant mortality rates. Cancers generally tend to be higher in the north-eastern industrial region of the USA, and so do heart attacks; but cancers of the cervix, uterus and skin tend in contrast to be high in the southern states, and in lower socio-economic groups. (Some standardized maps of cancers by counties are now available.)

Why are physicians where they are? There are the purely economic pull, the proximity to medical schools, the scale of facilities available, the attraction of metropolitan centres and especially of prosperous areas within them, the movement generally away from rural practices, and the effect of time-saving through easy access to hospital facilities on doctors' leisure time. There are some data about decision-making factors, and sub-optimal behaviour patterns prevail, largely because of conflicting goals—between professional commitment, economic motives, images of life styles in different locations and so on.

The evidence of the impact of geographic factors, especially distance, on health care, is more substantial, though studied in comparatively few areas. However, it is clear that the idea of 'distance decay' holds for many health care facilities—the concept that facilities will be proportionately more frequently used by populations nearer to a health centre, for instance, than by those at increasing distances from it (Figure 92). This may seem obvious, but a mathematical model, which has been subjected to computer analysis, will simulate the probability of populations at different distances from health facilities moving to use them.

Clearly this has potential in practice as soon as we think it possible that the spatial arrangements of hospitals and health centres could be rationally planned, not simply left to 'muddling

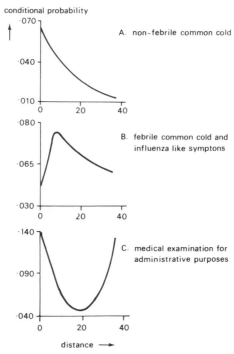

conditional probability

A. non-febrile common cold

B. febrile common cold and influenza like symptons

C. medical examination for administrative purposes

distance ⟶

Figure 92. Distance and use of health care: conditional probability of an individual consulting in a rural environment (based on work in Newfoundland). (Source: as Figure 86, Girt, J. L. in Shannon and Dever, Fig 5.1, p 99.)

through'. (It seems likely that other geographical approaches might well be applicable to locational and catchment area problems, including the whole field of network analysis.[6] Reilly's Law of 1931, originating in a study of retail marketing catchment areas in relation to populations of competing market cities, can be applied to health provision, while Jarvis's Law on the use of mental hospitals can claim a good deal of seniority, for it dates from 1851–52: 'The people in the vicinity of lunatic hospitals send more patients to them than those at a greater distance.'

This law can still be the basis for useful analyses, especially since a useful and much less obvious corollary can now be added: that the patients drawn from nearer populations also stand a much greater chance of resuming normal community life. Once enunciated, the reason behind the corollary may again be obvious but still worth saying: the patients will doubtless be drawn from a much wider spectrum of severity of affliction, or, conversely, distant patients must be hospitalized only when their disorder has exceeded a much higher threshold of tolerance for their families and friends. (On the other hand, Smith in 1976 suggests that patients from greater distances tend to be given more thorough treatment than easy-attendance ones living near the hospital.) There are clear practical implications for mental health planning, and mental patients after all make great demands on hospital beds. Distance decay can be shown to affect doctors' patterns of referral as well as patients' own behaviour. Thus in a study of perinatal mortality from Oxford, travel to consultant facilities of over 20 minutes reduced the referral rate from 60 to 50 per cent, while perinatal mortality was 18 per 1,000 for nearer patients and 21–2 per 1,000 for more distant ones.

Finally, methods are already available to forecast regional health developments, given a climate in which geographical inputs are used in health planning. For instance, the diffusion of a health care scheme in Detroit was analysed, allowing for an administrative limitation of the catchment area; this diffusion was then the subject of a simulation exercise, using the spatial application of the 'Monte Carlo' random diffusion model, as suggested by the Swedish geographer Hägerstrand.[7] Since the simulation was regarded as successful, there is the chance to forecast the rate of diffusion and direction of diffusion of future schemes of similar type and in similar cities; obviously there is potential applicability to practical problems in the future.

The work by Shannon and Dever is a pioneering synthesis on the geography of medical care, affording a great deal of stimulus to active participation on this frontier. However, many readers may find the issues crystallized by considering one more case study of rather a different kind from those discussed in Chapter 7.[8] Writing in 1970 Pyle was concerned to analyse the prevalence of morbidity or illness from heart disease, cancer and stroke in Chicago, in relation to ecological factors viewed in a particular and quite pointed way, and to project forward to 1980. First, he studied the morbidity from these causes and, second, the capacity of existing health service facilities to treat the patients and the areas where facilities would fall short of demand; he then followed through in a logical way to recommend optimal locations for additional hospitals and other facilities. Projection to 1980 seems a very short-term target, but this is a pioneering piece of work, of course building on earlier work. Thus in 1969 a method was devized to improve efficiency in allocating regional hospitals in Chicago.[9]

Pyle's study is in my view such an important piece of innovative thinking that it is well worth while examining for its methodology, rather than just for its contribution to health planning in Chicago, crucial though that may have proved. Crude morbidity and crude mortality rates were mapped, using 271 recording areas for the following data:

Name	International Classification
Total cardiovascular disease	400–468
Vascular lesions of CNS	330–334
Total cancer	
Cancer site groups	
*Digestive system	150–154
Respiratory system	162, 163
Genitals, male and female	171, 172–174, 177
Breast	170
Leukemia and aleukemia	204
Buccal cavity and pharynx	140–148
Skin	190, 191
All other and unspecified	196–197, 155–160
	164–165, 175–176
	178–181, 192, 195
	198–199

*Data for the seventy-five Chicago Community Areas include only rectum and large intestine.

The method used was trend surface analysis, a more mathematically sophisticated method of obtaining generalized spatial trends than my simple arithmetically derived 'generalized contours' of cancer in Victoria (Figure 47). It is unfortunate in relation to some possible uses of the maps that it was not possible to use standardized mortality ratios—as already noted, it is difficult to obtain data for them in the US—but for the main purposes the author had in mind the crude rates seem to have served their purpose. Several different mathematical formulae can be used for this process of spatial generalization, according to the characteristics of the particular set of 'hills and valleys' to be analysed, and it is not clear which particular method Pyle used.[10] Pairs of trend surface maps for 1960 and for 1967 give first indications of trends over time, as well as suggesting whether a spatial trend is consistent, and in that sense significant.

Figures 93 and 94 show the trend surface maps of heart disease; both maps show high rates in the city centre and in the suburbs. In contrast Figures 95 and 96, of strokes, show high rates in the city centre and in rural areas, and there is also a significant area of change in high rates along the north shore, coincident with middle-class residential expansion there. Figures 97 and 98 are for total cancers; these would be unsatisfactory for ecological analysis related to particular carcinogens or the like (which would need mapping for cancers of the lung, stomach etc separately), but they may be useful enough in projection of future needs in the way of cancer beds and diagnostic and treatment facilities—and, indeed, proved more useful from this point of view than did the mapping by cancer site.

As examples of the difficulties met in handling the cancer-by-site maps, consider Figures 99 and 100. While there are common elements in the two maps of cancer of the digestive system, the differences are too great to allow of useful forecasting. You may well agree with this judgement simply on comparing the two maps, but the methods of forecasting may throw further light on the problem, which may arise because the separate cancer-site maps are dealing with smaller numbers, where random fluctuations are affecting the patterns; or, as Pyle suggests, this problem may be compounded because a category like cancers of the digestive system on one classification includes cancers of ten sites within the gut, each with the possibility of distinctive aetiology and random fluctuations. Now the separate maps for cancer-sites are known to vary one from another more than do the individual types of heart disease from generalizations such as Figures 93 and 94, so, allowing for these fluctuations over time (admittedly only using 1960 and 1967 data), the problem may appear completely intractable. However, it proved that Figure 97 of total cancers

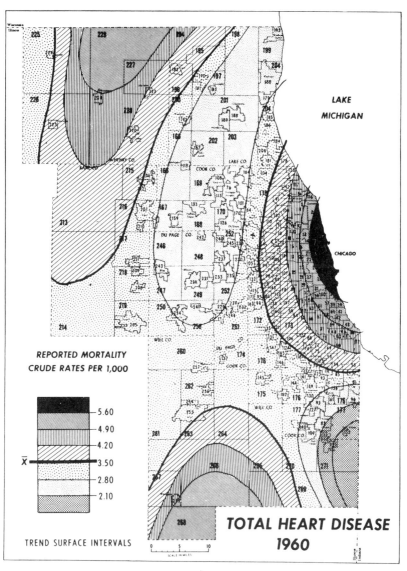

Figure 93. Chicago: total heart disease, 1960. (Source: Pyle, G. F. *Heart disease, cancer and stroke in Chicago: a geographical analysis with facilities, plans for 1980*, Chicago, University of Chicago, Department of Geography, Research Paper No 134, 1971, Fig 13, p 78.)

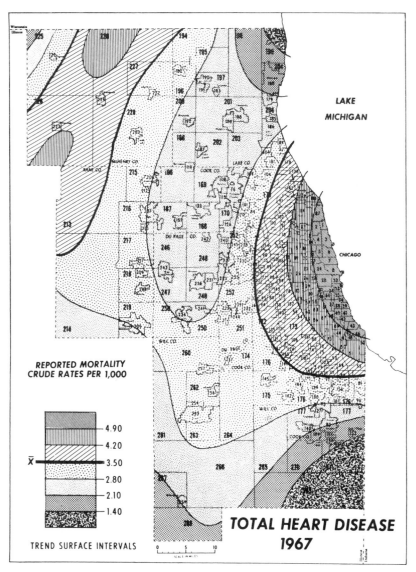

Figure 94. Chicago: total heart disease, 1967. (Source: as Figure 93, Pyle, Fig 14, p 79.)

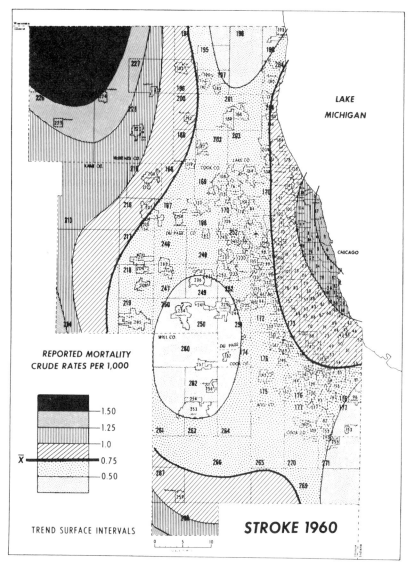

Figure 95. Chicago: stroke, 1960. (Source: as Figure 93, Pyle, Fig 15, p 80.)

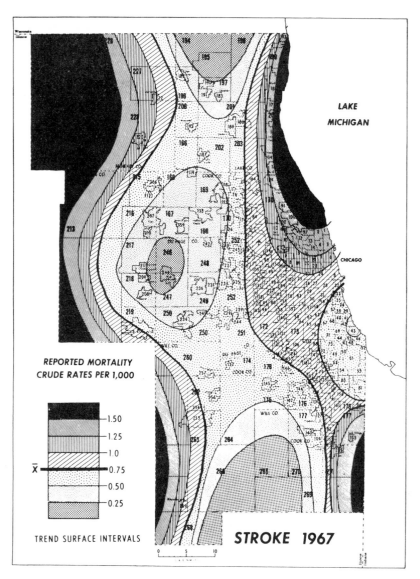

Figure 96. Chicago: stroke, 1967. (Source: as Figure 93, Pyle, Fig 16, p 81.)

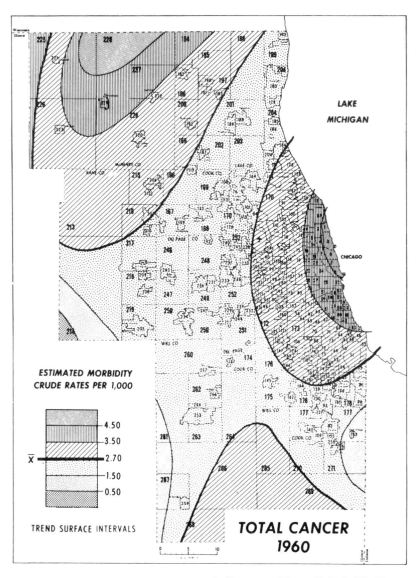

Figure 97. Chicago: total cancers, 1960. (Source: as Figure 93, Pyle, Fig 17, p 83.)

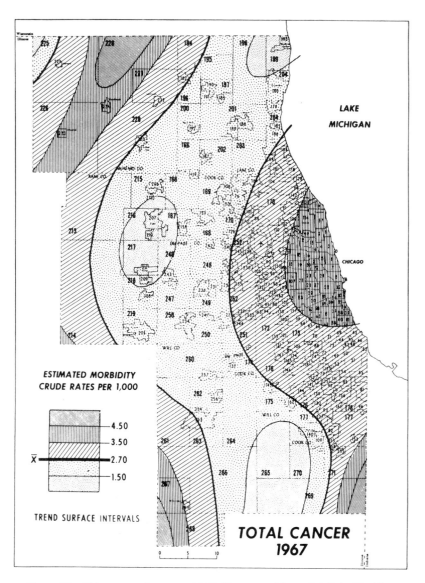

Figure 98.   Chicago: total cancers, 1967. (Source: as Figure 93, Pyle, Fig 18, p 84.)

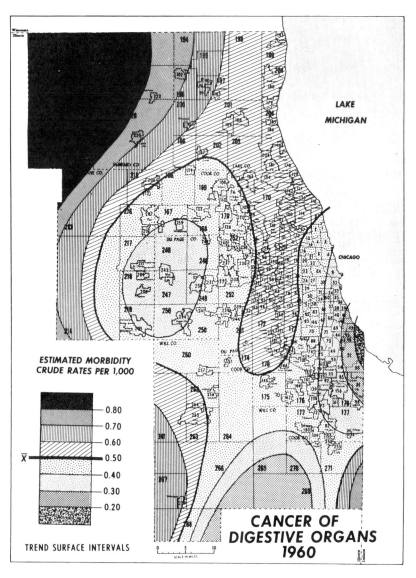

Figure 99. Chicago: cancer of digestive organs, 1960. (Source: as Figure 93, Pyle, Fig 20, p 86.)

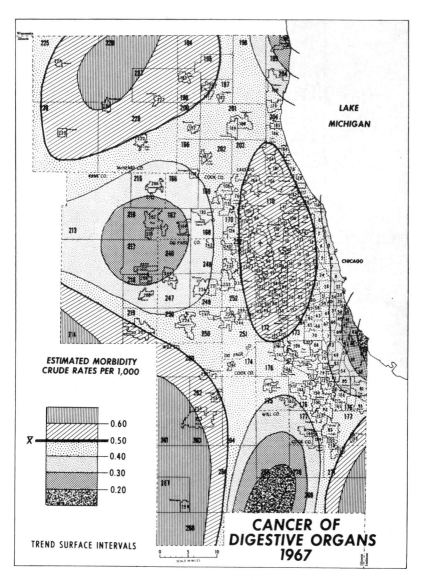

Figure 100. Chicago: cancer of digestive organs, 1967 (Source: as Figure 93, Pyle, Fig 21, p 87.)

provided a workable generalization of the individual site maps for broad analysis and projection. To quote: 'In other words, the sites tend to be spatially correlated much more with total cancer for respective temporal distributions than with each other over the seven-year gap.'[11]

Before moving on to the next stage of the analysis, note that breast cancers share this problem of temporal variation (Figures 101 and 102); however, the pattern is somewhat different and there is enough in common to be suggestive of higher incidence in better-class housing areas. Another contrasted pattern is that for leukemia (Figures 103 and 104); here the two maps do correspond fairly closely, and the pattern is suggestive of high rates in lower-income and especially black ghetto areas, where the general association of leukemia as a disease of young people correlates with high proportions of young age groups, and not necessarily with particular deprivations. If so, the maps may be more useful in forecasting than in aetiological speculation or analysis.

The next stage of the analysis was ecological in the sense in which the word ecology is often used in sociological and urban analysis. The morbidity and mortality data were subjected to a computer-based correlation exercise, in which each piece of disease data for the 271 recording districts was correlated with the following items also recorded for the same districts: population; population density; per cent substandard housing; per cent white-collar workers; average annual income; per cent unemployed; median education (the 'middle value' educational standard attained, using locally recognized yardsticks such as a certain level attained at school); population per household; per cent black; per cent foreign born; and age groups (each as per cent of community) of 0–15, 16–45, 46–65, and over 65 years. The aim was to discover if any of these items could be established as 'independent' variables, that is variables affecting the disease concerned. (If it does affect the disease incidence in a statistically significant way, the item can be used relevantly in a forecasting exercise even if the causal links between the socio-economic variable and the disease are not clear.)

This part of the work is based on the techniques of linear

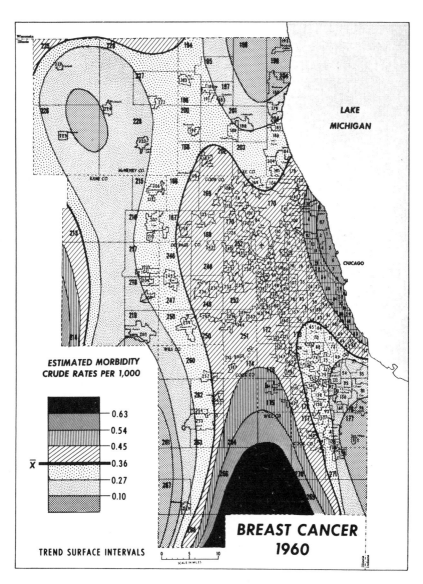

Figure 101. Chicago: breast cancer, 1960. (Source: as Figure 93, Pyle, Fig 26, p 95.)

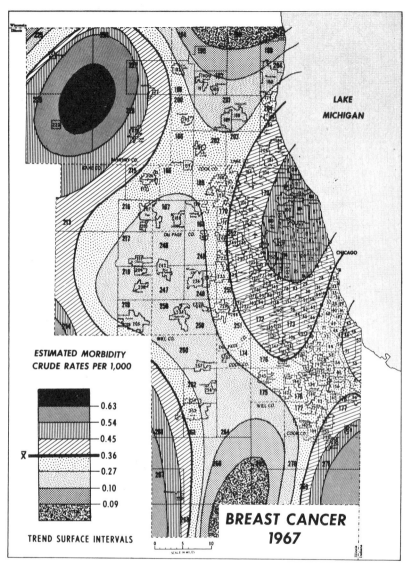

Figure 102. Chicago: breast cancer, 1967. (Source: as Figure 93, Pyle, Fig 27, p 96.)

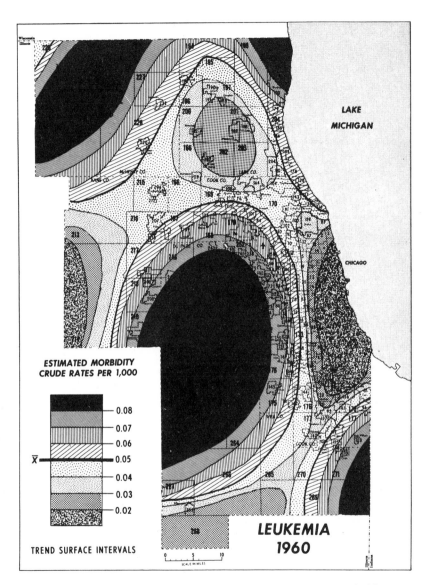

Figure 103. Chicago: leukemia, 1960. (Source: as Figure 93, Pyle, Fig 28, p 97.)

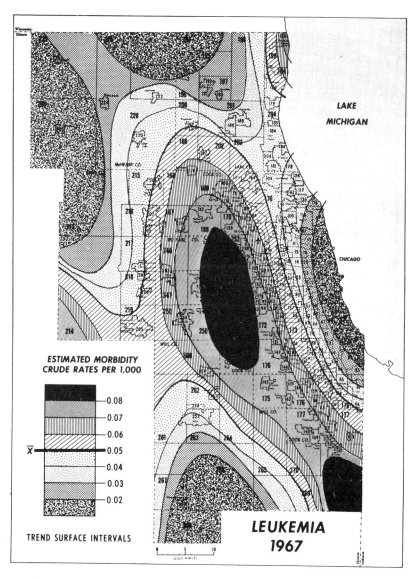

Figure 104. Chicago: leukemia, 1967. (Source: as Figure 93, Pyle, Fig 29, p 98.)

multiple regression analysis, and in particular on the method called path analysis by the geneticist Wright in 1960 (Figure 105). The essential in this method is to consider the ways in which a number of variables may conceivably operate upon each other as independent (apparently causal) variables or as dependent variables influenced by them. Of the various theoretical ways of linking the flow of influence, the most promising for further analysis appeared to be one in which a large number of variables seemed to influence a smaller number of 'key' variables (possibly with some interactions between these), which might be thought of as subsuming the effects of the original set.

The variables selected from the list above for this path analysis were population, density, income, per cent black and the four age groups. The findings themselves are not very surprising: the higher age groups are significant for heart disease, stroke and total cancers; the individual site data follow a similar pattern but with much weaker correlations—conformable with the previous indications that other factors were causing variations between the

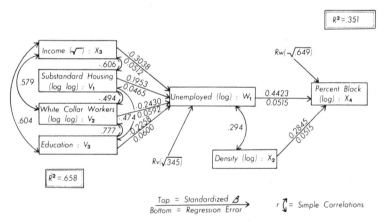

Figure 105. Chicago health care study: 'path diagram' of 1960 variables for a first alternative model, for regression analysis (ie statistical analysis of the extent to which variables vary together, one varying with another, whether in the same or opposite directions). This is simply a method of using logic concerning possible or likely relations between variables, in order to select likely 'paths' among the variables for analysis in search of correlations that may suggest causes (but not prove them, proof being a matter of actual observation of the causal process in some way). (Source: as Figure 93, Pyle, Fig 39, p 113.)

1960 and 1967 cancer site-maps, except for leukemia with its association with lower age groups and black and poorer areas. (Skin cancers showed quite a high correlation with higher income!) However, the point of the exercise was that for heart disease, strokes and total cancers it was possible to evolve equations for forecasting purposes; age over 65, population density and population play a leading part in all three equations.

This means that some of the maps in Figures 93 to 104 can be interpreted as maps of areas with high proportions of older people, in one sense. But if other evidence enables reasonable forecasting of the over-65s, the population density and the population—and other variables to a lesser degree in the three forecasting equations—then the need for hospital and other facilities can be forecast for the three disease categories mentioned—for heart diseases, for stroke and for total cancers. This is done for each of the three categories and similarly mapped by means of trend surfaces: (a) for crude mortality rates and (b) for number of deaths (each district covered by the belt between a certain pair of contours) perhaps the 200 and 250 contours, is expected to have, say, between 200 and 250 deaths. (The cancer data are mapped for morbidity rates and for cases, not mortality rates and deaths.) The next stage is to analyse the implications of the forecasts for provision of hospital and other facilities. It is at this point that the breadth and almost interdisciplinary quality of this study becomes clear.

Pyle analyses the cost-effectiveness of hospitals, which, like many organizations, tend to become more economical with size up to a point, then to become more expensive per unit of service. He does the same sort of analysis for such other facilities as x-ray and cobalt therapy, physiotherapy etc; and then analyses the 'distance decay' affect. Figure 106 illustrates the theoretical approach, and Figure 107 its application.

The study culminates in a series of 'iterations' or repetitions of a sequence of adjustments to the capacity of existing hospitals and other facilities, until they can no longer be further expanded economically. Then new facilities are added to the hospital provision, as for 1980, taking appropriate count of the distance decay in their location, and of the economies of scale for the particular

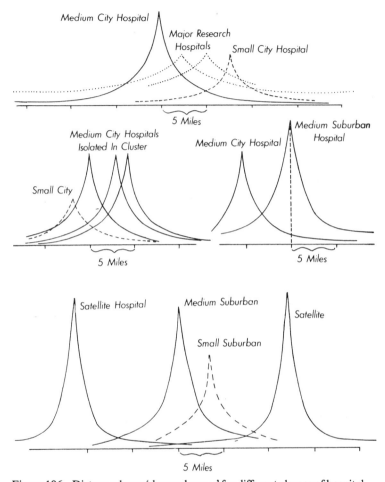

Figure 106. Distance decay 'demand cones' for different classes of hospital. These are simply graphs representing the fall in effective demand for the services of hospitals among the population at increasing distances from it. Thus in the top diagram the major research hospital spreads most widely its catchment area or the area in which it meets effective or actual demand, the medium city hospital commands a smaller catchment and the small city hospital a still smaller area. These graphs are referred to as cones because the different curves of distance and demand may be thought of as falling away from the hospital itself, not just in two directions, to right and left in the graph, but in all directions. To put the same idea more technically, the graph may be rotated, forming a sort of cone with curved surfaces, convex as one looks down on the resultant cone. (Source: as Figure 93, Pyle, Fig 51, p 147.)

238

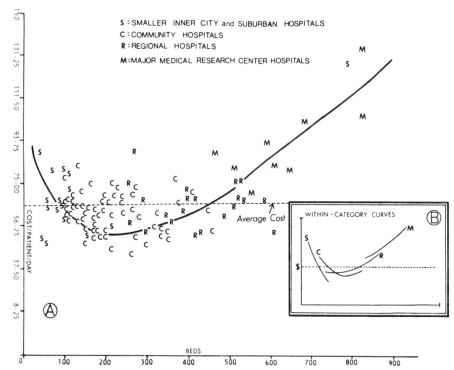

Figure 107. The Chicago hospital cost curve. This graph uses actual cost data from Chicago hospitals. Costs per patient are plotted on the graph for each hospital; their location on the graph are in relation to the cost scale on the vertical axis, while their positions are fixed by reference to the horizontal axis according to the number of beds. The index letters used for the various points plotted are for the different types of hospital noted on the diagram. The curved line is an expression of the general tendency for costs per patient to decrease as one moves from very small hospitals towards moderately large ones—the 'economies of scale' becoming effective—and then increase again as the hospital size rises above the economic optimum size. The inset shows that the curves vary somewhat for different types of hospital, and that clear indications of optimum size are only available for community and regional hospitals. (Source: as Figure 93, Pyle, Fig 54, p 155.)

type of facility in choosing their size. All but a small part of the 'unmet need' is met, and that is judged within the limits of error of the whole operation.

Pyle points out that the procedure, on existing techniques and knowledge, works best for cancers, despite the problem of different patterns for the several apparently distinct diseases by site that are included; this is attributed to its greater distinctiveness and ease of identification. The heart disease and stroke models were less precise and tended to overlap. Among his conclusions, Pyle points out how costly it would be if the projected increases in cancers, heart disease and stroke are to be adequately treated, even taking such a short run of years ahead as a decade. For instance, training programmes for many specialized personnel ought to be initiated at once, and budgeting for hospital provision begun. I write without knowing whether or not there has been a direct implementation of Pyle's model, or further more refined work intended to assist practical hospital planning. But whatever the answers to those questions, this is work of great significance for the methodology of the medical care side of the theme of this book.

Retrospect: two medical geographies or one?

It is clear that both the ecological medical geography of the earlier part of the book and this sort of geography of medical care have an important role in any country or community able and willing to plan its health services fundamentally. The ecological side, in the sense I have used the term through all the earlier chapters of the book, is of potential importance because aspects of the ecological web connected with human behaviour may well give the key to breaking a particular disease cycle, in a way complementary to the parasitologist's knowledge, or to the microbiologist's. Thus Prothero's work[12] on migration in Nigeria proved vital to malaria control programmes and complemented the work of malariologists, and this fresh light was thrown not on a newly discovered or newly evolved disease but concerned a cycle whose biology and therapeutics had been well enough known for decades and in some aspects for almost a century. The ecological side of medical geography must always be important because it may play its part, with sister sciences, in social, community or preventive medicine. Prevention is better than cure, and cheaper, but if cure there must be, then the rational planning of health services is vital, as is spatial analysis of the type illustrated in this chapter.

Some authors of papers on medical geography appear to lean

towards ecological medical geography, and this would apply to some writers choosing the term geographical pathology for their research. (I have written elsewhere of the contributions to medical geography from medical men and the medical sciences—much greater, so far, than that from the few medical geographers at work.[13]) Other authors lean towards health care geography. The most successful of the ecological school have seen their work applied in some small way in preventive medicine, the most effective method of health care where it can be accomplished. The health care geographers are by no means necessarily uninterested in medical ecology or in prevention, and in time may well spark off fresh ideas or investigations in these fields. The medical ecology workers tend to have their interdisciplinary links with the biomedical sciences, the health care geographers with demographers and economists, and possibly sociologists and social ecologists, and also to maintain strong links with current concerns in geography in general in quantitative, theoretical and applied aspects.

So far in western countries the two schools have maintained links in common, and one can claim that there is one medical geography. In the USSR my tentative impression is that only medical geography or nosogeography of various kinds is recognized as serious scientific endeavour; health care is left to the medical administrators of the comprehensive system and the hierarchy of Figure 88.

In health care geography there is often an assumption, implicit or occasionally explicit—and shared by some medical scientists of repute—that the great advances against infectious diseases have been made, and indeed such major advances as are likely in our time against cancers, circulatory breakdown, heart disease and the like. If this is indeed so, then the case for a very strong, even dominant, role for the health care as against the medical ecology wing of our field is unanswerable. However, in the world as a whole the amount of human misery and inefficiency caused by vectored and non-vectored infections is considerable, and the earlier chapters perhaps establish a claim that medical geography can throw light on contacts between man and the disease cycle, as indeed in Prothero's work just cited. Identification of a pathogen or even of the links in a disease cycle does not mean the end of problems of disease ecology or preventive medicine, or adjustment to living with the infection if that is the best approach. There does still seem to be a complementary role for both branches of medical geography.

Notes

CHAPTER ONE

1 Mahalanobis, P. C. and Das Gupta, A. 'The use of sample surveys in demographic studies in India', *Proceedings World Population Conference, Rome, 1954*, Papers, Vol 6 (New York, UN, 1955), 363–84

CHAPTER THREE

1 Vellar, O. D. 'Acute viral hepatitis in Norwegian track finders: an epidemiological study in Norway', *Acta Medica Scandinavia*, 176 (1964), 651–5
2 Pickles, W. N. 'Epidemiology in country practice', *New England Journal of Medicine*, 239 (1948), 419–27
3 Bailey, N. T. J. *The mathematical approach to biology and medicine* (Wiley, 1967), 182–210
4 Vols 43–50 (1968–75)
5 Say Vols 38–42 (1963–7)
6 Wingate, P. *The Penguin Medical Encyclopaedia* (Harmondsworth, 1972)
7 Hunter, J. M. and Young, J. 'Diffusion of influenza in England and Wales', *Annals of the Association of American Geographers*, 61 (1971), 627–53; also in McGlashan, N. D. (ed). *Medical geography: techniques and field studies* (Methuen/University Paperbacks, 1972)

CHAPTER FOUR

1 Bruce-Chwatt, L. J. 'Paleogenesis and paleo-epidemiology of primate malaria', *Bulletin WHO*, 32 (1965), 363–87
2 Learmonth, A. T. A. 'Some contrasts in the regional geography of

malaria in India and Pakistan', *Transactions of the Institute of British Geographers*, 23 (1957), 37–59

3   Prothero, R. M. *Migrants and malaria* (Longman, 1965)
4   Coles, Ann. 'Malaria in the Trucial States', *Institute of British Geographers Medical Geography Study Group Symposium, University of Strathclyde* (1972)
5   Fonaroff, L. S. 'Man and malaria in Trinidad: ecological perspectives of a changing health hazard', *Annals Association American Geographers*, 58 (1968), 526–56
6   Mann, Ida. *Culture, race, climate and eye disease: an introduction to the study of geographical ophthalmology* (Springfield, Illinois, C. C. Thomas, 1966), 373
7   Ibid, 159–60
8   Mann, op cit
9   T'ang, F. F., Chang, F. L., Huang, F. M. and Wang, K. G. *Chinese Medical Journal*, 75 (1957); see also Mann, op cit, 16
10 Stamp, L. D. *The geography of life and death* (Collins/Fontana, 1964)
11 Faber, London, 1962
12 Davey, T. H. and Lightbody, W. P. H. *The control of disease in the tropics* (H. K. Lewis, 1956)
13 Hunter, J. M. 'River blindness in Nangodi, Northern Ghana: a hypothesis of cyclical advance and retreat', *Geographical Review*, 56 (1966), 398–416
14 Ibid
15 Bradley, A. K. 'A case study of onchocerciasis in the Hawal Valley, Nigeria', WHO Mimeo WHO/OCHO/72.93
16 Ibid
17 Cockburn, A. *The Evolution and Eradication of Infectious Disease* (OUP, 1963)

CHAPTER FIVE

1   Allen-Price, E. D. 'Uneven distribution of cancer in West Devon with particular reference to the divers water supplies', *Lancet*, 1 (1960), 1235–8
2   Clemow, F. G. *The geography of disease* (CUP, 1903); Haviland, A. *The geographical distribution of disease in Great Britain* (Swan Sonnenschein, 1892)
3   Legon, C. D. 'A note on geographical variations in cancer mortality, with special reference to gastric cancers in Wales', *British Journal of Cancers*, 5 (1951), 175–9; and 'The aetiological significance of geographical variations in cancer mortality', *British Medical Journal*, 27 (1952), 700–2
4   Doll, R. and Hill, A. B. 'Lung cancer and other causes of death in

relation to smoking', *British Medical Journal*, 2 (1956), 1071–81

5   Stocks, P. 'Cancer and bronchitis mortality in relation to atmospheric deposit and smoke', *British Medical Journal* (1959), 74–9

6   Howe, G. M. (1963 and 1970)

7   Howe, G. M. *Man, environment and disease in Britain: a medical geography through the ages* (Newton Abbot, David & Charles, 1972), 55–6

8   Ibid, 234

9   Learmonth, A. T. A. and Nichols, G. C. 'Maps of some standardized mortality ratios for Australia, 1959–63', Department of Geography, Australian National University School of General Studies, *Occasional Papers*, No 3 (1965); Learmonth, A. T. A. and Grau, R. 'Maps of some standard mortality ratios for Australia, 1965–66, compared with 1959–63', ibid, *Occasional Papers*, No 8 (1969)

10   McGlashan, N. D., personal communication (1975)

11   Picheral, H. *Espace et santé: géographie médicale du Midi de la France* (Montpellier, Imprimerie du 'Paysan du Midi', 1976)

12   Cook, Paula and Burkitt, D. *An epidemiological study of seven malignant tumours in East Africa* (London, Medical Research Council, 1970)

13   Wingate, op cit, 77, 78–9, 148

14   Ibid, 78–9

15   Girt, J. L. 'Simple chronic bronchitis and urban ecological structure', in McGlashan, 1972 op cit

16   Howe, G. M. and Loraine, J. A. (eds). *Environmental medicine* (Heinemann Medical, 1974)

CHAPTER SIX

1   Picheral, op cit

2   After Aykroyd, W. R. *Conquests of deficiency diseases: achievements and prospects* (Geneva, WHO, 1970), 51

3   Cousens, S. H. 'The regional pattern of emigration during the great Irish famine, 1846–51', *Transactions of the Institute of British Geographers*, 28 (1960a), 119–34; and 'Regional death rates in Ireland during the great famine', *Population Studies*, 19 (1960b), 55–73

4   See the absorbing account in Cecil Woodham-Smith's *The great hunger*

5   Clark, C. *Population growth and land use* (Macmillan, 1967)

6   Aykroyd, op cit, and FAO/WHO/UNICEF Protein Advisory Group. *Lives in peril*, World Food Problems No 12 (Rome, FAO, 1970)

7   Dixon, B. *Invisible allies: microbes and man's future* (Temple Smith, 1976)
8   Flynn, M., Flynn, M., and Mellor, P. 'Social malaise research: a study in Liverpool', *Social Trends*, 3, 1972, 42–52
9   Wingate, op cit
10 Langer, P. 'History of goitre', *WHO* (1960), 9–25
11 WHO. *Endemic goitre*, WHO Monograph Series No 44 (Geneva, WHO, 1960); Kelly, F. C. and Snedden, W. W. 'Prevalence and geographical distribution of endemic goitre', *Bulletin WHO* (1960), 27–233; Howe and Loraine, op cit
12 McClelland, J. *Transactions of Medical Physiological Society*, 7 (Calcutta, 1835), 145; Stott, H. *et al.* 'Distribution and causes of endemic goitre in the U.P.', Part 1, *Indian Journal of Medical Research*, 18 (1930–1), 1059–85
13 Stott *et al*, op cit
14 See May, J. M. and McClellan, Donna L. *The ecology of malnutrition in seven countries of Southern Africa and in Portuguese Guinea* (New York, Hafner, 1971) and other works in the series.

CHAPTER SEVEN

1   Ffrench, G. E. and Hill, A. G. *Geomedical monograph series, regional studies in geographical medicine*, Vol 4, *Kuwait: urban and medical ecology. A geomedical study* (New York, Heidelberg, Berlin, Springer–Verlag, 1971)
2   Kanter, H. *Libya: a geomedical monograph* (Heidelberg Academy of Sciences, Berlin, Springer–Verlag, 1967)
3   Ibid, 146–9
4   Howe (1970), op cit
5   Coates, B. E. and Rawstron, E. M. *Regional variations in Britain: studies in social and economic geography* (Batsford, 1971)
6   Open University. *D203 Decision making in Britain*, Block 5, *Health* (Bletchley, Open University Press, 1972)
7   Shannon, G. W. and Dever, G. E. A. *Health care delivery: spatial perspectives* (New York, McGraw–Hill, 1974)

CHAPTER EIGHT

1   Shannon and Dever, op cit; Pyle, G. F. 'Heart disease, cancer and stroke in Chicago: a geographical analysis with facilities, plans for 1980', *Research Paper No 134* (Chicago, University of Chicago Department of Geography, 1971)
2   Shannon and Dever, op cit
3   Christaller, W. *Central Places in Southern Germany* (1933); trans

by Baskin, C. W. (New Jersey, Englewood Cliffs, Prentice–Hall, 1966)

4   Godlund, S. 'Population, regional hospitals, transportation facilities and regions: planning the location of regional hospitals in Sweden', *Lund Studies in Geography*, 21 (Lund, Gleerup, 1961)

5   Murray, M. A. 'The geography of death in the U.S. and the U.K.', *Annals Association of American Geographers*, 57 (1967), 301–14

6   See Haggett, P. and Chorley, R. J. *Network analysis in geography* (Arnold, 1969)

7   Hägerstrand, T. *Innovation diffusion as a spatial process*, trans by Ared, A. (Chicago, Chicago University Press, 1967)

8   Pyle, op cit

9   Morrill, R. L. and Earickson, R. J. 'Locational efficiency of Chicago area hospitals: an experimental model', *Health Services Research*, 4 (1969)

10 But see Haggett, P. *Locational analysis in human geography* (Arnold, 1965)

11 Pyle, op cit, 92

12 Prothero, op cit

13 Learmonth, A. T. A. 'Medicine in medical geography', in McGlashan, op cit (1972a), 17–42; and 'Atlases in medical geography', in McGlashan, op cit (1972b), 133–52

Bibliography

The two main abstracting journals, *Abstracts on Hygiene* and the *Tropical Disease Bulletin*, are the starting point for finding the many hundreds of articles that would have been cited in a more purely academic work. The reader wishing to follow up a particular topic or example will almost certainly be able to do so from them. I should also mention two indispensable guides—*Dorland's Illustrated Medical Dictionary* and Peter Wingate's *Penguin Medical Encyclopaedia* (listed in Notes). In conjunction with the sources in the Notes, the following books and papers should make up a useful reading list.

JOURNALS

Abstracts on Hygiene, monthly (Bureau of Hygiene and Tropical Diseases)

Tropical Disease Bulletin, monthly (Bureau of Hygiene and Tropical Diseases)

BOOKS AND PAPERS

Brownlea, A. A. *A medical geography of infectious hepatitis: ecological parameters in a system of Illawarra communities*, PhD thesis (Sydney, Macquarie University, 1969)

Burgess, E. W. 'The growth of the city: an introduction to a research project', in Park, R. E. (ed) *et al. The city* (Chicago UP, 1925)

Cooke, E. *Escherichia coli and man* (Edinburgh, Churchill–Livingston, 1974)

Defoe, D. *A tour through the whole island of Great Britain*, edited by Cole, G. D. H. and Browning, D. C. (Dent, 1974)

Doll, R. (ed). *Methods of geographical pathology* (Oxford, Blackwell, 1959)

Dorland's Illustrated Medical Dictionary (Philadelphia, W. B. Saunders)

248

Gregory, S. *Statistical methods and the geographer*, 2nd ed (Longman, 1963)

Holmes, J. 'Problems in location sampling', *Annals Association of American Geographers*, 57 (1967), 757–80

Houel, G. and Domadille, F. 'Twenty years of anti-malaria work in Morocco', *Bulletin of the Institute of Hygiene, Morocco*, 13 (1953), 3–51

Houel, G. 'Malaria control in rice growing areas of Morocco', *Bulletin of the Institute of Hygiene, Morocco*, 14 (1954), 43–90

Howe, G. M. 'Computers putting diseases on the map', *Nature*, 223 (1969), 891

Howe, G. M. 'Some aspects of social malaise in Scotland', *Health Bulletin*, 28 (1970), 1–23

Hoyt, H. *The structure and growth of residential neighbourhoods in American cities* (Washington, DC, Federal Housing Administration, 1939)

Hunter, J. M. (ed). 'The geography of health and disease', *Papers of the first Caroline Geographical Symposium (1974)*, Studies in Geography No 6 (University of North Carolina at Chapel Hill, Department of Geography, 1974)

Languillon, J. *et al.* 'Contribution à l'étude de l'épidemiologie du paludisme dans la région forestière du Cameroun. Paludométrie, espèces plasmodiales, anophelisme, transmission', *Médicine Tropicale*, 16 (Marseilles, 1956), 347–78

Learmonth, A. T. A. 'Geography and health in the tropical forest zone', in Miller, R. and Watson, J. W. *Geographical essays in memory of Alan G. Ogilvie* (Nelson, 1959)

McGlashan, N. D. (ed). *Medical Geography: techniques and field studies* (Methuen/University Paperbacks, 1972)

May, J. M. 'World atlas of diseases, No 15, World distribution of spirochetal diseases', *Geographical Review*, 45 (1955)

Ross, R. 'An application of the theory of probabilities to the study of *a priori* pathometry', Part 1, *Proceedings of the Royal Society*, Series A, 92 (1916), 204–30

Schaller, K. F. *Ethiopia: a geomedical monograph* (Heidelberg Academy of Sciences, Berlin, Springer-Verlag, 1972)

Snow, J. *On the mode of communication of cholera* or *Snow on cholera*, reprint of two papers (1849, 1855) by Snow, J., together with a biographical memoir by Richardson, B. W. and an introduction by Frost, W. H. (New York, the Commonwealth Fund, 1936)

Spate, O. H. K. and Learmonth, A. T. A. *India and Pakistan* (Methuen/University Paperbacks, 1967)

Acknowledgements

Acknowledgements are due and warmly made to the many people who have helped me in writing this book: to Ann Evans, who typed a difficult manuscript; to John Hunt, cartographer; to Professor Richard Lawton for much constructive criticism; to Dr J. B. Harley for thinking of me as a possible author and for patience in long delays; to Gillian Norman for a first suggestion concerning a book of this type and on the particular topic; to Valerie Cassidy for research assistance; to Alyson Learmonth for research assistance and some first drafts of chapters; and to Barbara Field for proofing.

The extracts from Dr P. Wingate's *Penguin Medical Encyclopaedia* are by permission of A. D. Peters & Co Ltd.

Sources of illustrations are acknowledged in the captions. I owe a particular debt to Professor G. M. Howe and the Royal Geographical Society for the many maps based on the *National Atlas of Disease Mortality*.

Index

The index does not include the names of authors whose work is cited in the chapter references, the bibliography, or acknowledged in captions to figures.